REJUVENATE

Mental acuity with everyday easy-to-follow cerebral challenges that literally exercise your brain, and by following Gary Null's sixteen rules of brain nutrition

RECOGNIZE

The foods, toxins, habits, and environmental factors that contribute to brain weakness

REVERSE

The effects of specific brain conditions such as headaches, depression, anxiety, memory loss, insomnia, senile dementia, and more

...THE NATURAL WAY, with this groundbreaking plan from America's foremost authority on quality natural living

classicalstretch.com

Chromium
zinc
magnesium
DHEA-S

Gary Null's

MIND

POWER

by GARY NULL

 NEW AMERICAN LIBRARY

New American Library
Published by New American Library, a division of
Penguin Group (USA) Inc., 375 Hudson Street,
New York, New York 10014, USA
Penguin Group (Canada), 90 Eglinton Avenue East, Suite 700, Toronto,
Ontario M4P 2Y3, Canada (a division of Pearson Penguin Canada Inc.)
Penguin Books Ltd., 80 Strand, London WC2R 0RL, England
Penguin Ireland, 25 St. Stephen's Green, Dublin 2,
Ireland (a division of Penguin Books Ltd.)
Penguin Group (Australia), 250 Camberwell Road, Camberwell, Victoria 3124,
Australia (a division of Pearson Australia Group Pty. Ltd.)
Penguin Books India Pvt. Ltd., 11 Community Centre, Panchsheel Park,
New Delhi - 110 017, India
Penguin Group (NZ), 67 Apollo Drive, Mairangi Bay,
Auckland 1311, New Zealand (a division of Pearson New Zealand Ltd.)
Penguin Books (South Africa) (Pty.) Ltd., 24 Sturdee Avenue,
Rosebank, Johannesburg 2196, South Africa

Penguin Books Ltd., Registered Offices:
80 Strand, London WC2R 0RL, England

Published by New American Library, a division of Penguin Group (USA) Inc. Previously published in a New American Library hardcover edition.

First New American Library Trade Paperback Printing, June 2007
10 9 8 7 6 5 4 3 2 1

The author expresses thanks for help with some of the recipes in this book to Marcus Guiliano from Aroma Thyme Bistro.

REGISTERED TRADEMARK—MARCA REGISTRADA

New American Library Trade Paperback ISBN: 978-0-451-21957-2

LIBRARY OF CONGRESS CATALOGING-IN-PUBLICATION DATA:
Null, Gary.
    [Mind power]
    Gary Null's mind power: rejuvenate your brain and memory naturally/by Gary Null.
        p.   cm.
    Includes bibliographical references.
    ISBN 0-451-21673-3 (hardcover)
    1. Memory disorders—Alternative treatment.   2. Brain.   I. Title.
    RC394.M46N85 2005
    616.85'2306—dc22   2005021658

Set in 11pt Ehrhardt

Printed in the United States of America

PUBLISHER'S NOTE
Every effort as been made to ensure that the information contained in this book is complete and accurate. However, neither the publisher nor the author is engaged in rendering professional advice or services to the individual reader. The ideas, procedures, and suggestions contained in this book are not intended as a substitute for consulting with your physician. All matters regarding your health require medical supervision. Neither the author nor the publisher shall be liable or responsible for any loss or damage allegedly arising from any information or suggestion in this book. The opinions expressed in this book represent the personal views of the author and not of the publisher.

In addition, the recipes contained in this book are to be followed exactly as written. The publisher is not responsible for your specific health or allergy needs that may require medical supervision. The publisher is not responsible for any adverse reactions to the recipes contained in this book.

Furthermore, the publisher does not have any control over and does not assume any responsibility for author or third-party Web sites or their content.

ACKNOWLEDGMENTS

For a seminal book of this magnitude, many months of constant, unrelenting research are required. I am grateful that I was able to assemble a top-notch team to assist me on this project. A very special thanks to Doug Henderson, Esq., and Jill Stern, for their invaluable, Herculean efforts in researching this material and in seeing this extremely important project through to its completion. Also, the efforts of Claire Zion and her assistant, Tina Brown, were crucial in navigating this project through waters that were, at times, turbulent. I'd like to also acknowledge the efforts of my literary agent, Mitchell Waters, who, once again, proved why he is the best agent in the world. And special thanks go out to Sondra Hollander, for her work in gathering the testimonials.

CONTENTS

PART III: APPENDICES

AN IMPORTANT NOTE ABOUT SUPPLEMENTS AND MULTIPLE CONDITIONS

This book is designed for individuals who have, or are specifically concerned about, only one of the conditions discussed below. To promote brain health and protect your brain, you should follow my protocol for optimal brain health in Chapter 2.

In the chapters that follow, I'll recommend protocols for specific conditions. The vitamins, minerals, and supplements I recommend should be incorporated into the protocol from Chapter 2. In some cases I will recommend increasing the dose of a particular vitamin or supplement to impact a specific condition. In these cases, you should increase the daily dosage from Chapter 2 to the level recommended for that specific condition.

Do not combine the protocols in these chapters with each other. And do not add more than one additional protocol to the one given in Chapter 2. If you are concerned about more than one of the brain conditions below, consult with a health professional about how you can safely impact multiple conditions. If you are taking medications, or have any food restrictions, you should consult with your doctor before beginning any supplement program. Supplement overdoses are rare, but possible, and certain combinations may affect individuals adversely.

PART I

UNDERSTANDING MIND POWER

INTRODUCTION

The dogmas of the quiet past are inadequate to the stormy present. The occasion is piled high with difficulty, and we must rise with the occasion. As our case is new, so we must think anew and act anew.

—Abraham Lincoln (1809–1865)

What does it mean to grow old today? The high-performing, result-oriented generation of baby boomers has entered middle age still determined to have it all. And in increasing numbers individuals are asking me: Does chronological age doom us to a sentence of gradual decline? Must we simply accept the inevitable weakening of our physical and mental powers?

My answer: Absolutely not. It is never too early—or too late—to change your lifestyle and behaviors to successfully maintain vigorous mental and physical health as you grow older.

In my book *Power Aging*, I proposed a proactive solution for people who wanted to take control of their bodies as they aged. I told those who would listen that growing older did not mean accepting the "inevitable" decline of aging—that they could fight the symptoms of aging and continue to feel young, and live life to the fullest. Thousands of people have followed this revolutionary program, making changes in their diets and lifestyles with astounding results.

Looking around me today, however, I still see the need for individuals—the baby boomers (born between the years 1946 and 1966)—to take control of their future health and well-being. And some individuals would claim that they are trying to do just that. They go to the gym, to yoga and Pilates; they follow one fad diet book after another. "Fifty is the new thirty," they claim, as they pop into their dermatologist for another shot of Botox.

But these measures result, at best, in some surface changes. They do not address the true needs of our aging minds and our bodies. And so, a vague feeling of uneasiness, perhaps even fear, continues to shadow us on our journey into middle age and beyond. As individuals in the boomer generation have become caretakers for elderly parents, or have seen relatives lost to the ravages of an age-related disease such as Alzheimer's, they begin to suspect that the surface changes they have made—their halfhearted attempts at a healthy lifestyle—are not enough. They want to know what they can do to ensure that they remain physically vigorous and mentally sharp.

In his seminal book *The Structure of Scientific Revolutions*, Thomas S. Kuhn secured his place as one of the most influential philosophers of science in the twentieth century. Significantly, his major contributions were not the result of his continuing the work of others, but of his breaking away from "the dogmas of the quiet past"—he was willing to look beyond positivist doctrines, those that emphasized only observable facts and excluded metaphysical speculation about the origins and causes of particular events, and in doing so, he gave birth to a new kind of scientific philosophy.

Before Kuhn, scientific knowledge was envisioned as an accumulation of all that had been learned over history, with each additional, newly discovered scientific law being piled onto the preceding facts. When Kuhn looked at science, however, he saw something entirely different. Instead of new laws simply being added onto the old ones and resulting in, at best, a small shift in the accepted body of knowledge, he believed science could be profoundly altered by the addition of each significant new discovery.

Kuhn envisioned a science as having, at any one time, a worldview, or a paradigm description of its environment. This scientific paradigm is a way of looking at and understanding everything that science holds—all of its laws, beliefs, procedures, and methods. Kuhn felt that most scientists participate in what they understand to be "normal science," which is any activity consistent with the existing scientific paradigm. Small gains are the rule, as small discoveries are stacked up as further evidence of the nature of the ruling paradigm. But, eventually, anomalies are bound to arise that the paradigm cannot resolve. As they do, some individual(s) may step out of the paradigm and propose some new principle or law to address this new anomaly. If the scientific community accepts the proposed change, then science experiences a paradigm shift, and science proceeds with a new view of reality and understanding of how the universe works.

What I am proposing is a similar paradigm shift in our perception of aging. Both my prior book, *Power Aging*, and now *Mind Power* are meant to explain the fundamental way in which our views, beliefs, and behavior must change.

Growing up in a small town in West Virginia in the 1950s and '60s, I was able to see several generations living together, and the importance of what happened when people went through transitions in life: adolescence, puberty, young adulthood, marriage, raising a family, and readjusting once the kids leave the house. Once a person hit fifty in my hometown, they were considered old. Nothing was really expected of them from then on, except that they were supposed to slow down and take it easy. Back then you weren't supposed to exercise after high school if you were a woman, or college if you were a man. You could support a Little League team or go to other sporting events, but that was always in support of someone you knew who was younger—a relative, more often than not—playing a sport.

Diets never changed. Everyone ate the same food every day. If it was Friday, you ate fish sticks. On Sunday, you would have pot roast after church. Your mother would put it on the stove to simmer early in the morning, so that when you got home it would be waiting for you. In the pot she would have all of the ingredients, including vegetables like string beans or broccoli. And after having cooked all day, when dinner was served it all looked the same: like some form of congealed mush. After eating, people wanted apple or lemon meringue pie or an upside-down cake, and they would have their coffee with sugar and cream.

As you had coffee, you would sit around the table and talk. You would talk about, more often than not, your aches and pains. You talked about your hormones bouncing off the walls when you were in your teens. You talked about having your whole life ahead of you when you were in your early or mid-twenties. You talked about your career in your thirties and how hard you were working to get to a point where you were secure. By the time you were in your forties, you talked about your teenagers, and you talked about your hemorrhoids. By your fifties you were probably talking about your arthritis and diabetes.

Once you were sixty, you were on a deathwatch—which meant that people were just happy you made it to sixty, because many people didn't. Then you were in your retirement. You were supposed to have a garden and play canasta or bridge once a week; you were supposed to be there to spend holidays with the family. And, of course, you were expected to turn out for the funerals of family and friends.

At any of these gatherings, conversations were short and to the point. "How you doing? Fine," and that was it. You didn't go any further. Because you either assumed it was none of your business, or didn't expect anyone was going to tell you anything you didn't know already. But everyone was presumed to be sick.

If you got to be seventy or seventy-five, you were considered to have hit a home run because you lasted so long. So if you died the next day, you had had a long, good life no matter how good the quality of your life actually had been—or how much you had suffered. It was all a numbers game. At no time did anyone ever consider that it was drinking coffee, smoking cigarettes, eating meat and trans-fatty acids, not exercising, being sedentary or being overweight that was contributing to people's ill health.

Today, my generation of baby boomers and our parents—those who are still alive—represent more than half of the American population. And you would think that with the number of wonderful, magnificent technological advances made from the time that I was a boy until today, we would have made more advances when it comes to public health. After all, we've developed laptops, cell phones, put men on the moon and explored the far reaches of space. But we have failed to provide for a means to vigorous, vital aging. We may have added a few years to the overall life span, extending a person's longevity, but we haven't done much for the *quality* of life.

The medical establishment tells us they are making great strides to improve the quality of life. With misplaced pride they tell us that we are in the midst of a war on cancer, a war on AIDS, a war on mental illness, a war on diabetes, a war on heart disease, and a war on arthritis.

In reality, what we are in the midst of is a medical Vietnam. This medical Vietnam produces 780,000 American casualties each year—people dying because of medicine. The number-one cause of death in America is bad medicine. Why do I say this? Because in the last fifty years there has been so little progress in preventing illnesses.

According to an article in *The Journal of Nutrition, Health and Aging*, by the year 2050, approximately 30 percent of people living in industrialized countries will be sixty-five years of age or older. That means that there will be an increase in neurodegenerative disorders that may cause considerable cognitive and physical impairment and shortened life span. And when we see someone like Bill Clinton with a coronary triple bypass operation, we must question how is it that none of his doctors noticed his health condition until it reached such a critical stage. The truth is that his health was allowed to deteriorate because the best doctors in America did not pay attention to his health until he had overt signs of heart failure. No one paid attention to Ronald Reagan until he was in the early stages of Alzheimer's disease. The same goes for Charlton Heston, Michael J. Fox, and Janet Reno—celebrities who have made us familiar with the diseases that have afflicted them. But never once did anyone ever say, "Could it have been anything that they did or didn't do that caused them to become sick?" Instead we all assumed they were doomed to their fates by their genes.

What I want to say to you about this is something crucial to the paradigm shift that I am proposing: *our genes can only be as healthful as the medium in which we allow them to exist.*

I speak with hundreds of people yearly about these concerns, and the one thing I've learned is that the greatest concern for most of the aging baby boomers is not so much the threat of heart disease, cancer, or even diabetes (which all have medical treatments of some kind). Rather, what people fear most is the loss of mental acuity. In particular, they fear that Alzheimer's, dementia, and Parkinson's are in their not-too-distant futures. As they age, they see a loss in their cognitive function—which is the loss in their ability to memorize and recognize. And they fear these early signs are sentences of doom.

Few people ask, "What is the cause of these age-related cognitive dysfunctions?" Were they to genuinely consider such a question, they would find the following causes: chronic inflammation, which damages both central and cerebral blood vessels; bad diet, which leads to nutritional deficiencies; hormone deficiencies; impaired breathing, which leads to decreased oxygen to the brain and impaired circulation; a deficiency in essential fatty acids (EFAs), which every brain cell requires; free radical damage; the adverse effects from prescription medicine; and damage from environmental pollution.

With an intelligent game plan, however, the baby boomers need not live in fear of mental decline. These conditions can be prevented and reversed with lifestyle modifications. It's an exercise in simple cause and effect.

This book is meant as a wake-up call, alerting you that everything in life is cause and effect. But we have been told about cause and effect by some truly brilliant minds: Hans Selye, who told us in the 1950s about the effects of stress, and Lawrence LeShan, who taught us in the 1960s that what we think, we then become, as well as many others.

But even as these minds shared their important discoveries with us, people still thought within the box. No paradigm shift occurred. As a result, the baby boomers are entering middle age and they don't know what to do. They know they don't want to look old and feel old. They don't want to retire. They know they still want a life. But they don't know how to get there. So many of them are, for the first time, doing something their parents never did. They are reinventing themselves. They are saying, "I'm not finished yet. I did what I was expected and told to do, and now I am going to do what I want to do. I am going to live the life that I deserve."

The time is ripe for a shift in the paradigm. In that context, we are seeing a transition. We are seeing a whole new generation of people who are not willing to wake up one day and have Alzheimer's, dementia, Parkinson's, ALS, forgetfulness, wrinkles, and arthritic joints. They are finally willing to stop long enough to say, "Cause and effect. If it works in finance, if it works in raising a child, it certainly should work with my body."

But the first step we have to take is a scary one, because before we can accomplish anything else we have to recognize that medicine does not use the best of science. Medicine has held on tightly to its current paradigm. Look at Vioxx, Celebrex, Ritalin, and Prozac. Look at the Dalkon Shield and DES. Look at all of the things that medicine has said would make things better. They have made things worse—far worse. And yet the medical community has continued on with no change in their protocols.

And yet all along, *science* has been saying that you can slow down the aging process. You can slow down and even prevent all diseases of the brain if you just pay attention to what you are putting into your body.

All along, science has said, "You are what you eat. The only material that can change you is what you give your body. So why would you give the cell, the DNA, the mitochondria something that would destroy, alter, or damage it?"

Science has told us we have approximately 65–100 trillion cells. And we know there are over 10,000 gene alterations per cell per day. The reason that our brains lose function as they age is because we damage them, rather than helping them repair themselves. Coffee, cigarettes, white bread, hot dogs, hamburgers, pizza, french fries, milk shakes, cheesecakes, pretzels and bagels, grilled cheese sandwiches, white rice, colas and candies—these are the things that allow for the biochemical reactions that cause inflammation, free radical damage, and glycation that end up destroying, harming, or altering the DNA. Such damage occurs all the time, and will continue to as long as we are doing nothing to change it.

But we don't have to "do nothing." As Director of Anti-Aging Research at the Institute of Applied Biology, I have reversed the aging process. I have increased the age span of rats by one-third by feeding them living foods, sprouts and green juices instead of little rat pellets. I was able to help human beings regrow hair where it had gone thin, balding, and gray. (And mind you, it was new hair with new color.) I was able to remove wrinkles and stop mental conditions from getting worse, improve macular degeneration, unblock arteries, knock out viruses like herpes and hepatitis, and rejuvenate the liver by stopping all negative input and replacing it with beneficial dietary and lifestyle habits. I was able to do this by utilizing the science of nutraceuticals—such as acetyl-L-carnitine, phosphatidylcholine, phosphatidylserine, and L-carnosine. I also used a lot of other nutrients. I used chlorophyll from the juices of fruits and vegetables, as well as phytonutrients from fruits and vegetables and their compounds and powders.

This is the future. This is what will allow a forty-year-old to look like a twenty-year-old and have the energy of an eighteen-year-old. This is what will allow seventy-year-olds to rejuvenate their brains so that their memories come back to what they were when they were at their brightest and sharpest. This is something we can achieve today, not in the next century. We don't need to wait for a patented, exclusive proprietary drug from a manufacturer. We can act today. But it takes a different commitment. It takes discipline, patience, and a desire to learn. It takes a paradigm shift in our understanding of health.

In preparing this book, we collected more than 545,000 studies in peer review journals just on vitamins and minerals alone. The studies described their biochemistry, their safety, and their efficacy. If you ask the average doctor, they are ignorant of nearly all of these studies. Few practicing physicians have time to keep up with even a tiny portion of new research. For instance, we know that by caloric restriction we can extend the life span. When is the last time your doctor told you to restrict calories? If you want to lose weight it's likely you'll be told to follow a high-protein diet that is high in calories—with all the inflammatory agents and by-products and estrogen stimulators that cause impotency and free testosterone reduction, which places a person in harm's way.

Our paradigm shift requires a new division of science. We need to create a public health science with public health practitioners—people specifically trained in the art and science of rejuvenation, detoxification, and utilization. Your physician has no background in this. We have to find a new way to bring these tools to the public.

This book is such a tool. It is specifically meant to help you understand what to do for your brain. In the end, this is not just about rejuvenating and protecting the brain as you age. It is about rejuvenating and protecting every cell of your body, with the brain being the primary focus. But everything you do for the brain will have residual positive impact.

When I go home now to see my family, almost everyone in my parents' generation is dead. And I think—my goodness, what killed all these people? Well, you could say that heart attacks, strokes, and diabetes killed them. But I say, "No. Their belief system killed them." Their inability to look at cause and effect killed them. Their lack of knowledge about appropriate lifestyle changes did them in. This is because the doctors and other health authorities in their lives didn't tell them what they could do differently and why they should. Hopefully, they will prove to be the last generation who believes without question everything their doctors tell them.

I look at the people I went to high school with and am shocked to see how sick they look. They look old and beaten up because they are living like their parents. They believe they are just doing what good citizens do. And indeed they all are good, decent, and kindhearted citizens, but they aren't good to themselves. And now all their illnesses and their prematurely aged bodies are a testament to what happens when you never question old beliefs.

And so, I challenge you to examine your definitions of aging, to challenge a belief system that tells you that you must accept a quiet decline, a gradual fading of mind, body, and spirit. I challenge you to remember that it is the quality of *your own* beliefs that ultimately determines the quality of your life and growth for your brain and your body, no matter what your age.

CHAPTER 1

YOUR AGING BRAIN

The brain is not, like the liver, heart and other internal organs, capable from the moment of birth of all the functions which it ever discharges; for while in common with them, it has certain duties for the exercise of which it is especially intended, its high character in man, as the organ of conscious life, the supreme instrument of his relations with the rest of nature, is developed only by a long and patient training.

—R. V. Pierce *(from* The People's Common Sense
Medical Advisor in Plain English, *1917)*

From the moment of conception, our brains are developing, growing, and changing, and scientists and researchers are constantly discovering new information about how our brains develop throughout our lives.

For instance, it had long been thought that the human brain created crucial neural pathways in the early years of life, then over the course of a lifetime worked to reinforce and strengthen the most important of these connections, while pruning away those that were underutilized. In other words, the brain was formed and influenced in early years, remained largely unchanged in middle years, and declined in old age.

Over the last few decades, as scientific research techniques have become more sophisticated, our ability to learn about the complexities of the brain has accelerated. Now scientists are discovering that the growth of the brain is far more complicated and ongoing than previously supposed. Studies have shown that crucial development in the prefrontal cortex occurs after the teen years, and other researchers have discovered that brain cells can continue to develop well into old age.

It is amazing to consider how our brains—these three-pound organs that constantly grow and change throughout our lives—are charged with the oversight of our entire being. This mass of tissue and nerves drives our intelligence, interprets input from our senses, initiates the movement of our limbs, and regulates the social aspects of our behavior.

In this chapter I will talk about the structure of the brain and how choices you make about your environment, lifestyle, nutrition, and other factors can impact the health of your brain as you age.

UNDERSTANDING THE BRAIN

To get the most out of the Mind Power program, you need to have some knowledge of the most basic structures and workings of the brain and to understand how external factors influence both the growth and decline of this amazing organ.

The Architecture of the Brain

Our brains sit under our scalps, within the bony safety of our skulls, floating in cerebrospinal fluid and covered by the *meninges*. The meninges consists of three layers: the *dura mater*, a thick membrane that can restrict the movement of the brain within the skull, preventing movements that may burst the blood vessels of the brain; the middle layer, or *arachnoid*; and the layer closest to the brain, the *pia mater*. Our brains are nourished by our circulatory system, converting the nutrients in our blood into fuel for the ongoing computations of its billions of nerve cells. The brain is covered with a thin layer of tissue called the *cerebral cortex*. This coating is also called gray matter because the nerves in this area lack the insulation that makes other parts of the brain appear white. Most information processing takes place in the cortex.

The Forebrain

When you look at a picture of the brain, it is likely that the first part you notice is the *cerebrum*. This intricate, wrinkled area, along with its covering, the cortex, is the source of higher-level functions. It holds memories, allows you to plan, imagine, and create. This is the part of your brain you use in problem solving, abstract thinking, and making judgments.

The cerebrum is split down the center by a deep fissure, creating two halves, each with very different functions. At the base of the split is a thick construct of nerve fibers called the *corpus callosum*, which keeps communication flowing between the halves of the brain. Signals from the brain cross over on their way to the body.

The right cerebral hemisphere controls primarily the left side of the body, and the left hemisphere controls primarily the right side of the body.

In most people the left hemisphere is dominant in controlling responses, as well as language production and understanding and cognitive functions.

The right side of your brain controls: temporal and spatial relations; pattern recognition; recognition of complex auditory tones; and communication of emotion.

Each of the cerebral hemispheres in the forebrain can be further divided into sections called *lobes*, which govern specific functions.

- **The frontal lobes** lie directly behind your forehead and control your ability to plan, reason, and imagine. They are also important in memory construction. The rear part of the frontal lobes has a motor area that controls voluntary movement. On the left frontal lobe, a section called *Broca's area* works to transform thoughts into words.
- **The parietal lobes** govern sensory combinations and comprehension of stimuli, such as touch, taste, temperature, and movement. The parietal lobes also function in reading and arithmetic.
- **The temporal lobes** are associated with music, memory, and sensation. These lobes also process emotion, including strong emotions such as fear. They are important in forming and retrieving memories.
- **The occipital lobes** process images from the eyes and link that information with images stored in memory.

The Midbrain

This area of the brain controls some reflex actions and is responsible for some voluntary movements.

The Hindbrain

The lowermost area of the brain is composed of the upper part of the spinal cord, the brain stem, and a wrinkled ball of tissue called the *cerebellum*. The hindbrain governs cardiac, respiratory, and vasomotor centers.

The Limbic System

Deep within the brain, hidden from view, lie the structures that make up the limbic system, the area of the brain that is responsible for our emotional states. These gatekeepers of the brain include:

- **The hypothalamus,** a structure the size of a pearl, which works as a regulator, returning your body's systems to a "set point." The hypothalamus controls hunger, thirst, response to pain, sexual satisfaction, as well as our emotions, such as anger, unhappiness, joy, and excitement.
- **The thalamus** acts as a clearinghouse for information flow between the cerebrum and the spinal cord. Clusters of nerve cells called *basal ganglia* surround the thalamus and are responsible for integrating movements.
- **The hippocampus** works as a memory indexer and is vital in the construction and reconstruction of memory.
- **The amygdala** regulates our stress responses to fear and anxiety.

Communication in the Brain

All of the structures in the brain communicate with each other and the rest of the body by sending signals through cells called neurons. Information passes from one neuron to another at a junction called a *synapse*. Chemicals known as *neurotransmitters* are released by one neuron, cross the synapse, and attach to a receptor in a neighboring cell. There are at least one hundred known neurotransmitters, all with individual chemical reactions that are occurring constantly at the millions of synaptic junctions in our brains.

Key neurotransmitters, which help the brain to function quickly and smoothly, include acetylcholine, serotonin, dopamine, glutamate, and GABA (gamma-aminobutyric acid). Maintaining the delicate balance of these neurotransmitters within the brain is crucial to brain health.

AGING AND THE BRAIN

Our brains begin to form just three weeks after conception and continue to develop, expand, and adapt throughout our lifetimes. Babies are born with over 100 billion neurons—roughly the same number they will always have. Over the next three years, trillions of synaptic connections are formed between these neurons. During this period of time, synapses that are frequently stimulated strengthen and proliferate, and synapses that are rarely used are discarded. Scientists use the term "plasticity" to define this period of adaptive growth.

Until rather recently, the prevailing theory has been that, from adolescence through adulthood and old age, the brain continues to simply discard neuronal connections. Doctors told elderly patients who were experiencing age-related conditions—such as memory loss and mental fatigue—that there was nothing they could do but accept the inevitable. "Old" neurons had died, and there were no new cells to replace them. A decline in mental sharpness was an inevitable by-product of aging.

But research has shown that our brain—this amazing organ that grows and learns through interacting with the world through both perception and action—can continually adapt and rewire itself. A Princeton research team has discovered that there is a natural regenerative mechanism in the mature brain that creates neurons that migrate to the cerebral cortex, where they "plug in" and become a new part of the brain's central circuitry.[1]

Think about the brain of an infant, which is constantly amassing new information and stimulation and enrichment for the neurons forming synaptic connections. Now consider your own perceptions about challenging your brain when you are middle-aged or during your elder years. Stimulation, mental activity, and challenge all are essential in brain growth and vitality. This new research brings new urgency to a key maxim for vigorous mental health at any age: "Use it or lose it!"

But clearly the issue of what weakens our brain function is not simply about the act of aging. Despite what we have been told for decades, we need not accept the idea that our bodies, or our brains, simply and inevitably "wear out" as we grow older. Staying vital both mentally and physically as we age requires paying close attention to the mind/body connection and the effects outside factors—such as environment, nutrition and diet, stress and emotion—bring to bear on our welfare.

NEGATIVE FACTORS AND BRAIN WEAKNESS

What does happen, as we grow older, is that we begin to experience the cumulative effects of negative lifestyle habits and outside influences. Mental health conditions that have been labeled "age-related" are more often the result of our neglect of our bodies *and* our brains. If we understand the negative factors and how they impact our mental vitality, we can make the changes necessary to ensure vigorous mental health throughout our lifetimes.

In the rest of this chapter I will discuss the key factors in your environment and lifestyle that can negatively impact your mental health as you age. In Chapter 3, you will find out how you can protect yourself from these external hazards and rejuvenate your brain naturally.

Environment and the Brain

Pollution and poisons in our environment are especially harmful to our brains. Here are the substances of greatest concern.

Toxic Substances

Our daily environment can be hazardous to the health of our brains. It is shocking to realize that there are approximately one thousand substances that may cause brain toxicity and accelerate the decline of the brain. Of these one thousand substances, there are several that we are in danger of being exposed to on a regular basis.

There are two main ways these substances cause brain damage:

- **Acute toxicity** occurs when there is a single exposure to high levels of a substance causing immediate neurological damage.
- **Chronic toxicity** results from continuous exposure to lower levels of a toxin and can result in long-term negative effects in the body.

There are four general categories of substances that may contribute to brain toxicity: heavy metals, solvents and fuels, pesticides, and carbon monoxide.

Heavy Metals

Heavy metals that are not metabolized by the body can accumulate in the soft tissue with toxic effect. Heavy metals enter our bodies through food, water, and air. They may also be absorbed through direct contact with our skin. Blood and urine tests can be used to assess levels of heavy metals in the body.

The list below contains four heavy metals that appear in the top ten substances on the 2003 Comprehensive Environmental Response, Compensation, and Liability Act (CERCLA) Priority List of Hazardous Substances, compiled by the Agency for Toxic Substances and Disease Registry (ATSDR).[2]

ARSENIC Arsenic is the most common cause of acute heavy metal poisoning in adults. Arsenic is released into the environment by certain manufacturing processes. It can be found in our soil, water, and air. The central nervous system, blood, kidneys, digestive system, and skin are the main targets of arsenic toxicity.

LEAD Children are particularly susceptible to lead toxicity because they are likely to ingest lead-containing substances, such as paint chips. (Paint manufactured prior to 1940 contains lead.) Lead exposure also occurs in the home as drinking water passes through pipes, drains, and soldering materials used on plumbing. Adverse effects of lead exposure occur in the brain, bones, blood, kidneys, and thyroid. A simple blood test can determine lead levels in your body.

MERCURY Mercury affects the cerebellum, the basal ganglia, and the visual centers of the occipital lobe. Among the many conditions linked to mercury in the body is short-term memory loss. Mercury is extremely toxic, and exposure can result in serious physical and neurological problems, and even death. Mercury is used in thermometers, thermostats, and dental amalgams. Mining operations and paper industries are significant producers of mercury. Until 1990, mercury was added to paint as a fungicide. Mercury is also present in the medicines Mercurochrome and Merthiolate, as well as in some childhood vaccines.

CADMIUM Cadmium is a by-product of mining and the smelting of zinc and lead. Fertilizers with cadmium are used in agriculture and may leach into water supplies. Cigarettes also contain cadmium. Inhalation or ingestion of cadmium can result in damage to the brain, liver, kidneys, bones, and lungs.

Other Toxic Metals

While not considered heavy metals, there are two other metals that pose serious dangers to the brain:

ALUMINUM We are exposed to aluminum in abundance. It is found in food additives, antiperspirants, drinking water, automobile exhaust, tobacco smoke, foil, cookware, cans, and ceramics. Researchers have discovered significant amounts of aluminum in the brain tissues of patients with Alzheimer's disease. Although there is no conclusive evidence either for or against aluminum as a factor in Alzheimer's disease, research continues into the relationship between aluminum and such serious brain conditions as dementia and Alzheimer's.

MANGANESE Manganese toxicity is a well-recognized hazard for those who may inhale manganese dust. Inhaled manganese is transported directly to the brain, and may cause neurological symptoms similar to those of Parkinson's disease. The symptoms of manganese toxicity generally appear slowly, over a period of months or years. Used in gasoline as an antiknock additive, the manganese-containing compound MMT was approved for use in the United States in 1995. Manganese may also be ingested by drinking contaminated water, and may also cause neurological symptoms.

Solvents and Fuels

Paints, glues, and thinners contain substances that have been shown to cause neurological problems. The usual symptoms of persons exposed to these toxins include fatigue, headache, and confusion.

TOLUENE Toluene has been associated with long-term neurological problems, such as dementia, balancing and coordination problems, as well as brain atrophy. Toluene occurs naturally as a component of crude oil and is produced in petroleum refining and coke oven operations. It can also be found in gasoline. Do not be lulled into thinking you have escaped its ravaging effects once you are inside your home, however, for toluene can be found in household aerosols, nail polish, paints, and cleaning agents containing a solvent base.

Sniffing or "huffing" substances containing toluene on a continual basis causes permanent brain damage. Researchers have long studied how exposure to solvents has affected humans. Among the deleterious effects are a wide variety of brain conditions, such as cognition, attention, and memory problems. Depression and anxiety have also been associated with exposure to solvents.

Pesticides

In my research I have seen numerous varieties of pesticides that have neurotoxic effects on humans. When exposed to pesticides, a person may develop headaches, fuzzy vision, and have difficulty speaking. In severe cases, the lungs or other organs may fail. The main ways in which a person is exposed to pesticides are through inhaling its gases or absorbing the chemical through the skin.

Carbon Monoxide

Carbon monoxide is invisible, odorless, tasteless, and kills like a silent assassin. Unlike other toxic gases that emit noxious fumes, carbon monoxide is odorless, so people can unknowingly be exposed to its vapors and will become unconscious, and often die, due to a lack of oxygen to the brain. During the last decade, carbon monoxide poisoning has made big headlines in the United States. But until the deaths of high-profile individuals—such as tennis star Vitas Gerulaitis—from carbon monoxide poisoning, the importance of carbon monoxide detectors was on the back burner. Now, laws in many states mandate that each home be equipped with carbon monoxide detectors.

When carbon monoxide does not kill, it wreaks havoc on the brain, causing memory loss and other cognitive impairments. The hippocampus, a part of the brain vital for creating new memories, is especially vulnerable to the effects of carbon monoxide.

Lifestyle and the Brain

Just as your external environment can influence the health and welfare of your brain, your internal environment, the way you react to events and emotions, has an equally powerful impact on your mental health. Our daily behaviors and habits, if unexamined and unchanged, can predispose us to suffer some of the serious health conditions associated with aging.

Stress

Much has been written about how stress affects the brain. For instance, according to the National Institute of Mental Health, stress and depression are closely linked. A recent study shows that stress can actually rewire the emotional circuits of the brain.[3] Stress is not only psychological, but also physiological—in fact, stress can actually destroy nerve connections.

Specifically, constant stress produces disproportionate cortisol levels in the brain. Cortisol is a hormone that is released from the adrenal glands in response to a physical or psychological threat. When cortisol is continually produced, it will begin to impair the function of the hippocampus, the area of the brain that is related to memory. High cortisol levels from excessive stress result in atrophy and death of the neurons, destroying brain cells in the hippocampus and frequently affecting short-term memory.

In his book *Does Stress Damage the Brain? Understanding Trauma-Related Disorders from a Neurological Perspective*, J. Douglas Bremner, an Emory University professor of psychiatry and radiology, has used his more than ten years of research as a clinical psychiatrist to explain how changes in the brain that are the result of stress may be the cause of some psychiatric disorders, including, among others, depression and anxiety.[4]

According to a report from Stanford University, intense stress may even cause brain damage that leads to major depression or eventual memory impairment. In an article written for the journal *Science*, Stanford researcher and professor Robert Sapolsky discusses what science has learned so far about how stress adversely impacts our bodies.

Sapolsky cites a number of studies: one that looked at the hippocampi (the part of the brain responsible for explicit, declarative memory) of people who had recovered from long-term, major depression, another that studied Vietnam veterans, and a third that measured the left hippocampus of adults who suffered from post-traumatic stress disorder because of childhood sexual abuse. In all of the studies, the hippocampi in these severely stressed individuals were smaller than those in the control groups.[5]

In his book *Why Zebras Don't Get Ulcers*, Sapolsky emphasizes how stress adversely affects our whole bodies. Once stress triggers the sympathetic nervous system, hormones are secreted and a whole host of physiological changes occur that prepare the body for (what it perceives to be) impending danger.[6] This response is obviously beneficial to us when, for instance, being pursued by a tiger, but it also suppresses the immune system. Constant exposure to this type of stress and the resulting suppression of the immune system opens the door for many diseases, both physical and mental.

Unhealthy Habits

There may be some daily habits that you indulge in that damage your brain. And remember, habits that you recognize as being unhealthy for your body are just as damaging to your brain as those that you may indulge in without full knowledge of the risks.

NICOTINE Despite the well-advertised adverse effects of tobacco, nearly 25 percent of the world's population smokes cigarettes. While most people understand the link between smoking and cancer or heart disease, few are aware of the fact that the effects of nicotine on the brain are equally as dire. Cigarettes lower oxygen levels in the blood, and studies have shown that chronic smoking decreases blood flow to the brain. Nicotine prompts brain cells to grow nicotinic receptors—cells that respond to the neurotransmitter acetylcholine. This rush of acetylcholine explains why smokers may feel energized and clearheaded.

But as acetylcholine production continues at an unnatural rate, the delicate balance of neurotransmitters in the brain is upset and mental sharpness begins to suffer. This is particularly noticeable for anyone who has undergone the symptoms of nicotine withdrawal, which the American Psychiatric Association classifies as a mental disorder.[7]

ALCOHOL The negative effects of alcohol on the body are generally obvious. Alcohol consumption hastens the breakdown of antioxidants, negatively impacts the central nervous system, inhibits vitamin absorption— leading to liver damage—and is toxic at a cellular level. The effects of alcohol on the functioning of the brain are also far-reaching, negatively influencing areas involved in emotion, processing sensory information, and regulating stress. Alcohol disrupts the balance of key neurotransmitters, including serotonin, endorphins, and acetylcholine. Evidence also suggests that alcohol can alter the activity in the hippocampus, a part of the brain that is vital in memory. Alcohol acts as a depressant, decreasing the activity of the nervous system.

CAFFEINE Excess consumption of caffeine can wreak havoc with sleep patterns, deplete the body of critical B vitamins, upset the stomach, as well as cause physical symptoms such as tremors and exacerbate anxiety. Withdrawal from this potent drug is associated with irritability, headaches, depression, and nervousness.

Inactivity

Back in the day, people used to believe that as we age we should slow down, take it easy, and accept that our bodies can no longer keep up with an active lifestyle. This prescription for physical inactivity is, in fact, the worst possible advice for both your body and your brain.

A sedentary physical lifestyle contributes to impaired cardiac and respiratory systems, diabetes, arthritis, obesity, high blood pressure, osteoporosis, and insomnia. A sedentary mental lifestyle can lead to anxiety, depression, memory loss, and loss of cognitive function.

The mind/body connection is particularly clear when it comes to the connection between being both mentally and physically active. Muscle activity and chemical activity in the brain are closely related. In fact, bodywork practitioners find that deep muscle massage often triggers the release and awareness of powerful memories and emotions. Neurotransmitters such as acetylcholine and dopamine work to regulate muscle movement and fine motor skills, and in return, muscle activity serves to stimulate and increase synaptic receptors.

The benefits of physical exercise on the brain are many: improved blood flow, increased oxygen, and the release of mood-regulating neurotransmitters. The benefits of mental exercise are equally impressive: stronger neural connections, stimulation of new neuron growth, balanced levels of neurotransmitters, and increased memory and cognitive functions.

There is no reason to let any of your muscles—including your mental muscles—atrophy simply because you are getting older. An active lifestyle with an active interest in stimulating and enriching activities is a key component in keeping our brains vital as we age.

Nutrition and the Brain

Poor nutrition and an inadequate diet are leading causes of many brain-related diseases and conditions that are often attributed solely to aging. Most Americans fuel their bodies and brains with fast food, refined carbohydrates, trans fats, and sugar. Those who think they are eating more healthfully don't consider the fact that they are consuming meats, fruits, and vegetables that have been genetically modified, irradiated, or raised in toxic environments where earth and water may be contaminated with pesticides and fertilizers.

While I have spent a great deal of time and effort working with people to educate them about the effects of poor nutrition on their bodies, I now feel that I have to speak out just as strongly about the damage their diets and way of living are doing to their brains. According to Dr. Joel Fuhrman, who specializes in treating illness through nutrition and is the author of *Fasting and Eating for Health*, the frightening fact is that our American diet literally causes our brain to shrink, by depriving it of necessary nutrients and oxygen over the course of our lives.[8]

In the next chapter I talk about nutritional and lifestyle solutions that will protect your brain over a lifetime. But before you move on to reading about my Mind Power Nutritional Plan for Optimum Brain Health, you should fully understand the damage you are doing to your body, and thus your mind, by following the diet of the average American. When considering what you put into your body, you should know that your brain health is compromised by the consumption of sugar and fats and by a lack of vitamins and minerals.

Sugar

Sugar is high on my list of substances that should be completely banned from our diets. Sugar is nothing short of toxic to our bodies, yet Americans consume, on average, 140 to 160 pounds of sugar each year. Sucrose, or refined sugar, is quite different from glucose, the fuel that your brain needs to operate smoothly. Glucose is a simple sugar that is obtained from the metabolism of carbohydrates in foods and circulates through the bloodstream to provide the body with energy. Meanwhile, refined sugars challenge the immune system, causing diabetes, hypoglycemia, tooth decay, and obesity, to name only a few conditions. Sugar depletes B vitamins and calcium, and generates exceptionally high levels of cell-damaging free radicals, promoting inflammation throughout the body, especially in the brain. Overconsumption of sugar savagely attacks metabolism, causing a wide range of symptoms, including irritability, anxiety, confusion, nervousness, mood swings, lack of concentration, fatigue, depression, and headaches.

Fats

High-protein diets have been promoted, especially in recent years, as a quick way to lose weight. These diets preach what the average American wants to hear: you can eat lots of cholesterol and lots of saturated fats and lots of animal protein and still lose weight. Weigh these dietary tips against the fact that heart attacks and strokes kill about 50 percent of all Americans, and the connection is clear: the standard Western diet promotes cardiovascular disease.

As cholesterol and fats are transported through the bloodstream to the delicate tissues of the brain, the cells in the brain become coated with a waxy substance. This amyloidal protein buildup, or plaque, is found in the brains of individuals suffering from Alzheimer's disease. This amyloidal plaque has an inflammatory effect on the brain tissue. Inflammation is a prime cause of brain aging; I discuss it in more detail below.

There is no doubt that high-fat diets have an adverse effect on the entire circulatory system, but you may not recognize how this directly impacts the brain's health. As plaque buildup narrows arteries and tiny blood vessels (arteriosclerosis), the flow of blood throughout the body—and to the brain—is slowed. Blood that does reach the brain is oxygen-poor and lacking in nutrients, literally causing brain cells to die and the very mass of the brain to shrink.

Even as fewer nutrients are reaching the brain as a result of a high-fat diet, there is still more damage being done. Saturated fatty acids interfere with glucose use in the brain, starving the brain of energy and impairing cognitive function.

Vitamin and Mineral Deficiencies

A diet that relies on refined carbohydrates, sugars, and animal proteins as its building blocks does not leave a lot of room for taking in important nutrients from plant products. The healthy brain needs B vitamins—especially B_6 and B_{12}—as well as folate, vitamins E and C, and zinc. Nearly all of these important nutrients can be found in plant-based products. And few Americans are getting enough of them in their daily diets.

Special Risks

In addition to environmental, lifestyle, and diet factors, there are two other causes that play a significant role in brain aging.

Brain Inflammation

Inflammation is the body's response to stress, disease, and injury. It is the hallmark of every chronic disease. While the inflammatory response is a sign that the body's immune system is functioning and vital, when it is too strong or does not naturally suppress itself, it becomes damaging.

Inflammation of the brain plays a prominent role in Alzheimer's and dementia. The hippocampus, the region of the brain closely linked to memory, seems to be particularly vulnerable to neuroinflammation. Blood and urine tests can show whether markers of inflammation are elevated.

Hormone Imbalance

Hormones are natural chemicals that are produced in one location in the body and transported, via the bloodstream, to signal other organs or systems in the body. In short, they are responsible for the functioning of the trillions of cells in the human body. When any one hormone falls out of balance, the entire communication system in the body breaks down.

With aging, changes naturally occur in the level of hormones and the body's response to them. It is important to maintain a balance of hormones in the body to protect the brain against changes that may lead to depression, anxiety, or decreased cognitive functions.

SUMMARY

After you have read this chapter, I hope you can see how easy it is to practice a lifestyle that creates a healthy environment for your brain. When you ignore the health of your body, you are just as effectively ignoring the health of your brain. Just like your body, your brain doesn't have to become fragile or weak simply because it is growing older. The good news is that it is possible to make changes to create a healthy environment for your mind.

In the next chapter I will show you a diet and supplement plan, as well as lifestyle practices, that will protect your brain and even reverse the impact that negative behaviors, habits, and environments have had up to this point.

In Part 2 of this book, I will discuss specific conditions and diseases of the brain, such as depression, mental fatigue, senile dementia, and Parkinson's disease, and show you how to naturally fight their debilitating symptoms.

It is never too late to implement these changes. The brain is a remarkable, adaptable, and regenerating organ. Given the right environment, the right nutrition, and proper stimulation, it will thrive, regardless of its chronological age. By making a concerted effort to make the positive changes I discuss in the next chapter, you can set the stage for optimal performance from both your mind and your body, and discard notions of inevitable and "age-appropriate" mental and physical decline.

CHAPTER 2

PROMOTING AND PROTECTING BRAIN HEALTH

For even the mind depends so much on the temperament and disposition of the bodily organs that if it is possible to find some means of making men in general wiser and more skillful than they have been up till now, I believe we must look for it in medicine. It is true that medicine as currently practiced does not contain much of any significant use; but without intending to disparage it, I am sure there is no one, even among its practitioners, who would not admit that all we know in medicine is almost nothing in comparison with what remains to be known, and that we might free ourselves from innumerable diseases, both of the body and of the mind, and perhaps even from the infirmity of old age, if we had sufficient knowledge of their causes and of all the remedies that nature has provided.

—René Descartes (1596–1650), Discourse on Method (1637)

Aging successfully in both mind and body requires us to attend to all aspects of our lives: to embrace new challenges, to exercise limbs and cognition, to promote emotional health, and to provide our brains and bodies with the fuel that will allow them to grow healthily from infancy through old age.

In this chapter I will discuss the basic and fundamental strategies for maintaining brain health. Think of this chapter as the overview for having a healthy brain. *Everyone* needs to follow this advice. In later chapters in Part 2, I'll discuss strategies tailored to specific disorders of the brain that only those of you with special concerns will want to follow.

But first we all need to follow the advice in this chapter. I will offer you ways to continue to stimulate your brain, ensuring that neuronal pathways remain strong and productive. I will touch on the role of exercise in keeping both the body and the mind healthy, and how nurturing healthy social and emotional relationships benefits our minds as we age. Finally, I will discuss optimal diet and nutritional habits and give you a plan of foods, vitamins, and supplements that is your first line of defense against age-related mental decline.

LIFESTYLE HABITS FOR A HEALTHY BRAIN

The way we choose to live can have a huge effect on brain health in the long and short term. Here are the crucial areas of our lives that can contribute.

Challenge Your Brain

Research has documented that the brain requires constant stimulation and challenge to develop to its fullest potential. From studies that stress the importance of stimulation in a child's first three years of life,[1] to those that show how using your five physical senses and your emotional sense in unexpected ways will strengthen, preserve, and grow brain cells, science has proven again and again that we must "use it or lose it." In an article published in the *St. Petersburg Times*, the Pittsburgh neurologist Paul Nussbaum, speaking at the joint meeting of the National Council on Aging and the American Society on Aging, stressed that specific training for the brain, such as learning sign language, can boost IQ and promote a lifetime of brain growth, which, if continued, can stave off dementia and other brain diseases as people age. Other brain-challenging activities include taking up a second language, learning to knit, practicing public speaking, or learning to play a musical instrument.[2]

Lawrence C. Katz, Ph.D., a professor of neurobiology at Duke University Medical Center and the coauthor of *Keep Your Brain Alive: 83 Neurobic Exercises*,[3] suggests a series of exercises that can easily be done on a daily basis and involve one or more senses in a novel way. This type of "cross-training for your brain" can help keep your mind fit to meet any challenge.

Try some of the following ways to challenge your brain:

- Use your nondominant hand to go through your morning rituals of hair styling, toothbrushing, and makeup application.
- Shower with your eyes closed, using your tactile senses to adjust water temperature and flow and your sense of smell to locate shampoo and soap.
- With your eyes closed, locate your house keys and open the door to your home.
- Turn a photo album upside down and study the pictures.
- Shop at a new grocery store.
- Read part of the newspaper or a book upside down.
- Sleep on the other side of your bed.

The good news is that, young or old, we can continue to learn. The more complex the learning challenge, the more we stimulate our brains and the more vital they remain. Travel, reading, going to museums, and attending book-group readings all contribute to an active brain life. So play Scrabble, or do crossword puzzles, or enjoy bingo, or learn a foreign language. Growing older does not mean we should lose our sense of curiosity in the world around us, or our desire to pursue new challenges.

Exercise Your Body

Most of us know that physical exertion is good for our bodies. But it is also essential for our brains. Exercise should be a natural part of your life, whatever your age. If you do not exercise on a regular basis, or feel that you are too old to embark on a physical fitness program, you can begin to build a stronger body and brain by the simple act of taking a walk. Studies show that senior citizens who walk regularly show significant improvement in memory skills compared to sedentary elderly people. Walking can also improve learning ability, concentration, and abstract reasoning.[4]

Another long-term study that tracked a group of older men and women with no signs of dementia over a seven-year period found that those with a high participation in leisure activities, including walking or participating in an exercise class, were 38 percent less likely than others in the study to develop dementia.[5]

In still another study on physical activity and its effects on brain health, researchers at the University of California in San Francisco measured the brain function of nearly six thousand women during an eight-year period. The results were then correlated with the women's normal activity levels. The study showed that no matter how much or how little the women did in terms of exercise, there was a direct correlation to cognitive performance. It wasn't simply a matter of all or nothing. For every extra mile walked per week, there was a 13 percent less chance of cognitive decline.[6]

But walking is not your only choice. Citing a 2003 study published in the *New England Journal of Medicine* that showed that ballroom dancing at least twice a week made people less likely to develop dementia, the AARP (American Association of Retired Persons) recommends dancing as one of the best mind/body workouts.[7] Researchers speculate that the combination of learning and remembering specific steps and sequences specifically boosts brain power.

Looking for a sport that is easier on your muscles than dancing or walking? Advocates of the gentle, controlled movements of tai chi claim the significant benefits of stress reductions and improved balance and muscle tone. The memorization of specific movements and sequences is similar to learning new steps to a gentle and serene dance.

There is no doubt that even the most basic exercise offers our bodies and our brains long-term benefits. Dr. Kristine Yaffe, Chief of Geriatric Psychiatry at the San Francisco Veterans Administration Medical Center, estimated the protective effects of regular activity against cognitive decline could be as high as 40 percent.[8]

Whether you choose to walk, or dance, or garden, or practice tai chi or yoga, the most important thing is to get your body moving. The effects of physical activity are beneficial in delaying the onset of dementia, preventing the development of Alzheimer's disease, and improving memory and reasoning skills. Exercise also acts as a powerful antidepressant. No matter how old you are, it is never too late to experience the powerful benefits of some kind of physical activity.

Begin slowly if you must, but attempt to work up to forty-five minutes of exercise at least five days per week.

Strengthen Your Spirit

As we grow older, we can experience a sense of isolation and perhaps feel like withdrawing from interaction in society. This type of shutting down—of emotion, intellect, or spirit—is as unhealthy for our brains as the more easily recognized damaging habits of poor diet or lack of exercise.

Numerous studies have shown that individuals who have a strong sense of purpose and meaning in their lives thrive in their later years. Frequent contact with family and friends, participating in one's community, and feeling satisfied with one's accomplishments are key in maintaining mental health.

A positive outlook and ongoing social and emotional involvement are essential in keeping our brains stimulated and vital as we age. Ursula Lehr, Ph.D., of the University of Heidelberg and the former secretary of health of the Federal Republic of Germany, states that many studies have found that people who are mentally active—have a wider range of interests, farther-reaching perspectives, and a greater number of social contacts—reach old age with greater feelings of psychophysical well-being.[9]

Practicing meditation may be valuable for brain health as well. In a recent article published in the *Washington Post* online edition, Dr. Richard Davidson, a neuroscientist at the University of Wisconsin, discussed the findings of a study conducted over the past few years evaluating the effects of meditation on Tibetan monks. The results of the study demonstrate, according to Dr. Davidson, that ". . . the brain is capable of being trained and physically modified in ways few people can imagine."[10]

When the monks' brains were measured by MRI, Davidson found that the ones who were the most accomplished practitioners of meditation had brain waves that were better organized and coordinated compared to those of novices who had not been practicing meditation for as long. The more years spent meditating, the higher the gamma wave activity. In previous studies, mental activities such as focus, memory, learning, and consciousness were associated with this kind of high-level neural coordination.[11]

Research in this area is ongoing, but I have no doubt that meditation can be a powerful tool in promoting a healthy brain.

NUTRITION FOR A HEALTHY BRAIN

In this section I will give you a nutritional plan that you can follow to ensure that your brain is protected as you age. This basic plan provides the diet and supplements that our bodies need to fuel its cells—including those in the brain—for optimal performance and health.

This eating plan is simple, easy to follow, and nonrestrictive. I don't want you to think of this approach to healthy eating as a "diet." Diets can leave you feeling deprived and lacking in energy. Diets tend to focus on a goal of weight loss, rather than an overall enhancement of health. They can rob your body of essential nutrients and food groups and put you on the road to bad food habits. While you may lose weight when you follow my protocol for a healthy brain and body, what is more important is what you will gain: energy, focus, and mental vitality.

The supplements have been chosen specifically for their beneficial effect on brain function and health, but you will notice other health benefits as well.

Of course, before you begin any new health program, you should get a comprehensive, full-body evaluation performed by a qualified health care practitioner. A proper health and medical evaluation should evaluate your blood chemistry to assess your blood markers, your metabolic rate, and your blood pressure for indicators of cardiovascular, hormonal, or other imbalances or danger signs. If you are taking medications of any sort, you need to inform your doctor of any supplements you are considering adding to your daily diet, as some may interact with prescription medications.

The Nutritional Plan

Let's start with a discussion of what to eat.

Complex Carbohydrates

Complex carbohydrates are the gold standard when it comes to brain foods. They are the starches and fibers in foods like whole grains, nuts, tubers, beans, seeds, lentils, fresh fruit, and vegetables. Incorporate these foods into your diet in place of refined white rice, pasta, and bread.

To maximize the nutritional benefits of complex carbohydrates, you should eat them in whole food form. For many years, I have recommended that you eat five or more servings of organic fruits and vegetables each day. You should especially choose dark green, leafy, and root vegetables, like broccoli, watercress, carrots, sweet potatoes, brussels sprouts, spinach, green beans, or peppers—either raw or lightly cooked. You should select fresh fruits, like apples, berries, citrus fruit, pears, and melon.

In addition, you should consume at least four servings of whole grain foods, such as oats, rice, rye, whole wheat, millet, corn, or quinoa in cereal, breads, and pasta. Remember, when you can, to also include the skins of fruits and vegetables. Fruits and vegetables are excellent sources of fiber.

You may wonder, "Gary, how can fiber help my brain?" Well, fiber helps lower cholesterol and blood pressure levels, which are linked to Alzheimer's disease, as well as other degenerative brain diseases.

A NOTE ABOUT SUGAR Carbohydrate sugar converts to glucose, and, as such, is indispensable to the health of our brains, but one should try to obtain it in as pure a form as possible. Eliminate all refined sugar from your diet. This is not quite as easy as it may sound, for sugar is a hidden ingredient, lurking in many processed foods. We all know sugar can be found in soda, candy, and cakes. But how many of us know that it is also in bread, breakfast cereals, condiments, cheeses, and canned foods? I am fully aware that eliminating sugar from your diet will not be easy. You need to read the nutritional labels on processed foods. It will be worth the effort.

But don't make the mistake of thinking that a quick candy bar is fueling your brain. Common table sugar has been processed to 99.9 percent sucrose, which is stripped of the vitamins and minerals found in sugar cane or sugar beets. The refined sucrose taxes the body's digestive system, depleting it of essential vitamins and minerals and enzymes as the sugar is metabolized. For this and other reasons, white sugar is known as an "empty food." Choose whole grain carbohydrates as your body's source of glucose.

Fruits and Vegetables

Fruits and vegetables are packed with the essential vitamins and protective antioxidants that promote optimal brain function. Eating a wide variety of organic fruits and vegetables is crucial to a brain-healthy diet.

ANTIOXIDANTS Free radicals, atoms with unpaired electrons that can cause damage (oxidation) in the normal metabolic process, are an important factor in the aging process. Brain cells are particularly vulnerable to oxidation because of their high-energy production. They are constantly firing messages back and forth. As more energy is produced, a greater number of damaging free radicals occur. The destructive effects of the free radical process have been implicated in conditions such as Alzheimer's and Parkinson's disease.

But here's some good news: Two studies out of the University of South Florida Center for Aging and Brain Repair reinforce evidence that specific fruits and vegetables may guard against the brain being ravaged by free radicals as you age.

"If these pre-clinical findings translate to humans, it suggests that eating a diet high in antioxidant-rich fruits and vegetables may help reverse declines in learning and memory as you get older," said Paula Bickford, Ph.D., a professor at the University of San Francisco Center for Aging and Brain Repair, and the lead author of the two studies.

The first study involved feeding older rats a diet with high amounts of spinach over a period of six weeks. The results showed a reversal in the normal loss of learning that occurs with age. As noted above, spinach is a great source of antioxidants.

The second study concerned the value of a diet high in fruits and vegetables. The results found that the benefit of such a diet depends on the amount of antioxidants contained in the fruits and vegetables. The researchers imply that the protective effects of antioxidants may be connected to their ability to reverse the havoc caused by inflammations in the brain. Dr. Bickford found the greatest benefit in richly colored fruits and vegetables, which have the highest antioxidant levels. She recommends having spinach salads for lunch and snacks of blueberries and strawberries.[12]

Antioxidants, which work to protect the cells against free radical damage, are naturally occurring in many fruits and vegetables. Eating these beneficial foods essentially detoxifies the brain, ridding it of free radicals. Antioxidants include vitamins E and C, alpha-lipoic acid, grape seed extract, and coenzyme Q10. Antioxidants are especially found in the following foods: apples, berries (blueberries, raspberries, blackberries, strawberries), cherries, cooked kale, cranberries, garlic, grapes, prunes, raisins, and raw spinach.

ORGANIC PRODUCE All fruits and vegetables you eat should be organic, whenever possible, and there is certain produce that is especially risky. According to the Environmental Working Group (EWG), a nonprofit environmental watchdog agency based in Washington, D.C., eating the twelve most contaminated fruits and vegetables would expose a person to nearly twenty pesticides per day on the average. The EWG lists the twelve most contaminated fruits and vegetables on its Web site (www.foodnews .org/reportcard.php):

- apples
- celery
- cherries
- imported grapes

- nectarines
- peaches
- pears
- potatoes
- red raspberries
- spinach
- strawberries
- sweet bell peppers

The Web site also lists the twelve least contaminated fruits and vegetables:

- asparagus
- avocado
- bananas
- broccoli
- cauliflower
- kiwi
- mango
- onion
- papaya
- peas
- pineapple
- sweet corn

To these lists I would add leafy greens, since we consume the part of the plant that is sprayed, and nuts and seeds, such as almonds, pumpkin seeds, walnuts, sesame and sunflower seeds, which, because of their oils (which are beneficial), can hold chemicals for longer periods of time.

Washing fresh produce may help reduce pesticide residues, but it does not eliminate them entirely. Peeling reduces exposure, but valuable nutrients are also lost along with the peel. If you cannot buy organic produce, then choose foods from the least-contaminated list, and be sure to wash all fruits and vegetables thoroughly before eating them or using them in recipes.

Proteins
Most people are under the impression that you must have animal proteins in order to sustain life. This is a myth perpetuated by the meat industry. Consequently, we have given vegetables, grains, nuts, seeds, fruits, and

herbs a nutritional backseat, or relegated them to being an insignificant accompaniment, or garnish, to a meat-based or animal protein–based diet. This idea was the result of propaganda and marketing, though it was scientifically inaccurate.

In point of fact, my own original work with Dr. Hillard Fitsky and Dr. Victor Berman at the Institute of Applied Biology showed that virtually all foods contain all eight essential amino acids, and that we have been led to believe that only animal foods contain these amino acids.

We must make sure that we are receiving high-quality amino acids— nine-tenths of a gram per kilogram of body weight, which is approximately fifty grams per day for women and seventy grams per day for men. (Pregnancy, lactation, recovery from various illnesses, surgery, and infection will require more.)

The best foods for high-quality protein from fiber sources are grains (millet, buckwheat, brown rice, spelt, rye, quinoa, oats), legumes, nuts, seeds, tofu, tempeh, and fatty deepwater fish (such as cod, tuna, sole, salmon, and sardines). Good vegetable sources include yams, potatoes, sweet potatoes, gourds, squashes, and cruciferous vegetables (such as broccoli, cabbage, cauliflower, onions, asparagus, mustard sprouts, and sea vegetables, as well as soy and rice protein shakes).

Keep in mind that protein digestion is greatly improved by using the proper cooking techniques. By moderately heating most proteins, you increase their digestibility. This is especially true when dealing with beans, grains, and meat. Beans and other legumes contain several toxins that become nontoxic when cooked or sprouted.

Fats

Our bodies and brains need fat to function. But there are harmful fats and good fats. Making informed choices about the types of fat in the foods you eat is important in the proper feeding of your brain.

We all know the saturated fats in fried foods and the trans fats in processed foods should be avoided. But let's talk about the good fats that we should be sure to include in our diets.

Eating nuts and seeds (the best choices are pumpkin, sunflower, hemp, flax and sesame, walnuts, almonds, pine nuts, pistachio seeds, and chia seeds) provides beneficial amounts of intelligent fat for your brain. To increase the nutritional benefit from these seeds, you can grind them before using them in your meals.

Einstein considered fish to be brain food. And this is no fish tale. He was right. Your brain will love you if you eat cold-water fish—salmon, mackerel, herring, and fresh tuna. Consuming cold-water fish three times per week supplies your body with good amounts of the ever-important omega-3 fatty acids. Omega-3 fatty acids are known to benefit patients with chronic inflammatory diseases, including cardiovascular disease and arthritis.[13] The benefit of omega-3 fatty acids may help reverse brain damage resulting from chronic inflammation that is linked to aging and degenerative diseases. Another benefit of omega-3 fatty acids is that they prevent blood from clotting too rapidly, which could improve cerebral functioning by increasing cerebral blood flow.[14] A study conducted by researchers from the Department of Veterans Affairs (VA) and the University of California at Los Angeles (UCLA) found that a diet high in docosahexaenoic acid (DHA)—an omega-3 found in relatively high concentrations in cold-water fish—dramatically slowed the progression of Alzheimer's disease in mice. Omega-3 fatty acid supplements are now being tested in clinical trials with early-stage Alzheimer's patients in the United States, Canada, and Sweden.[15] By fighting plaque buildup in the arteries, fish improves blood flow to the brain and helps lower the risks of heart disease and stroke. Choose fish that is caught in the wild—not farmed. Studies have shown that farm-raised fish have high levels of toxins in their flesh.

There are even more benefits to omega-3 fats and other essential fatty acids (EFAs) called omega-6s. EFAs serve as building blocks for nerve cells and membranes. Our brains consist almost entirely of fatty acids. Without an adequate level of EFAs, dangerous saturated fats will take their place in cell membranes. Saturated fats reduce membrane fluidity and efficiency, thereby contributing to premature aging and disease development. Deficiencies in fatty acids have been linked to chronic inflammatory conditions, such as arthritis, hypertension, memory loss, dementia, cardiovascular disease, and insulin resistance (leading to Type II diabetes).

Foods high in EFAs include salmon, mackerel, sardines, herring, flax oil, walnuts, oysters, and tuna.

Just as there are fats that are beneficial to your brain, so there are fats that are clearly harmful to your brain. Saturated fats are very unhealthy. Excess saturated fat is linked to the increased likelihood of cardiovascular disease. Relative to all of the other fats, saturated fat is the most damaging. Saturated fats wreak havoc on blood vessels and interfere with blood circulation. They increase the production of LDL cholesterol (the "bad" cholesterol), which increases blood cholesterol levels, thereby increasing the risk of heart disease.

You should avoid consuming foods that are high in saturated fats—with the exception of raw and organic coconut oil—including sunflower and corn oils, which are commonly found in processed foods like salad dressings, french fries, pastry, and the majority of margarines, and hydrogenated vegetable oils found in processed foods like boxed cakes, microwave popcorn, and TV dinners.

Sixteen Rules of Nutrition

So far in this chapter I have outlined the general principles of healthful nutrition to help protect your aging brain. This program is good for all of us, and the more closely you follow it the more you will strengthen your brain. Even before you experience problems, you should follow these programs. They are preventive, too.

The more you incorporate these recommendations into your eating habits, the better off you are. Some of us can only manage to follow some of these guidelines. Others start with baby steps, and as they feel better they want to do more.

For those of you who want to do everything you can to change your nutritional intake to strengthen your brain, I have included the following sixteen rules for best brain health. Even if you can't follow all these guidelines, you'll be better off than if you take none of the advice in this chapter. But those of you who can keep to the sixteen rules all the time will be best of all.

1. Eat no animal meat or shellfish. Replace them with cold-water fish, such as wild salmon, trout, mackerel, sardines, cod, and sea bass, four to six times a week.
2. Eat nuts and nut butters, such as almond butter and walnuts, as well as sunflower seeds, pumpkin seeds, chia seeds, and sesame seeds.
3. Eat soybeans and soy products.
4. Eat whole grains, such as quinoa, amaranth, spelt, and teff. Include beans (of which there are over seventy varieties commonly available, from black-eye peas, navy beans, adzuki beans, lentils, split peas, and lima beans, to turtle beans).
5. Eat no dairy, including milk, yogurt, cheese, butter, ice cream, or cream sauces. Replace them with rice milk, soy milk, almond milk,

or oat milk. Do not use any nondairy product with casein in the ingredients.

6. Use no caffeine or alcohol. This means cutting out chocolate, coffee, tea, wines, hard liquor, and beer. Replace them with decaffeinated herbal teas and grain beverages, such as Postum, Cafix, Raj's lemon water, or green tea (which has small amounts of caffeine but also has threonine, which neutralizes caffeine and has a very beneficial calming effect).

7. Eat no sugar or artificial sweeteners. Replace them with stevia root, raw unfiltered honey, molasses, brown rice syrup, or natural food sweeteners. You can also use chromium picolinate—200 mcg—to curb sugar cravings.

8. Use no carbonated beverages, including sodas or seltzer. Replace them with spring water, distilled water, filtered water, or fresh-squeezed organic juices.

9. Eat no processed bread or wheat products. Replace them with spelt bread, sprouted whole grain breads, rice bread, or Essene bread. Make sure to *read the labels* to ensure they do not have refined flours, sugars, or trans fats.

10. Eat only certified organic produce. This applies to all vegetables, fruits, beans, grains, legumes, nuts, seeds, and potatoes.

11. Eat no deep-fried or processed foods. Replace them with sautéed, steamed, stir-fried, or broiled meals.

12. Use brain-healthy oils for cooking, such as macadamia and safflower oils. For baking, use hazelnut, macadamia-coconut, or mustard seed oils. For salads, use walnut, flax seed, or extra-virgin cold-pressed olive oil.

13. Eat no food additives, preservatives, coloring agents, flavorings, or MSG.

14. Eat no bedtime snacks. Eat primarily during the day. Try to have your largest meal between one and three p.m., a light breakfast, and a very light dinner.

15. Avoid dehydration. Make sure you drink plenty of fluids throughout the day. It's important not to lose our liquid balance, because then we will upset our electrolyte balance, our lymphatic balance, and our cleansing and elimination program. Most people should have a minimum of a gallon of water per day, but if you are sweating profusely or exercising vigorously, perhaps more is needed. It

is best to have an impedance test, which will determine what percent of your body is water. Ideally it should be between 72 and 74 percent, because for each percentage under that you will be losing your body energy and lessening the process of cleansing and detoxification. Liquids can include purified water or juices, plus one or two cups of green tea daily, lemon juice to help alkalize the body, and digestive enzymes to help with the tea.

16. Make no excuses. Keep a positive outlook and be sure to appreciate how your body and brain begin to feel and act younger after just a short time following this protocol. Commit to healthy living habits and maintain them for the sake of your long-term mental and physical health.

The Supplement Plan

In addition to choosing fresh, organic foods and using brain-healthy ways to prepare them, it is possible to further boost the health of our brains by supplementing our daily menu of foods with vitamins, minerals, and other supplements that specifically target and enrich the function of the brain.

In truth, it can be hard to get the optimal levels of the vitamins and minerals we need through diet alone. Although the nutrients we get from foods are more powerful, we should ensure we are getting adequate quantities by taking supplements as well—to complement (not substitute for) our healthful eating habits.

Vitamins and Minerals

VITAMIN B COMPLEX The B vitamins play an important role in promoting brain health. One study reported that middle-aged men who had the highest amounts of vitamin B_6 in their blood scored best on memory tasks as compared to other middle-aged men who had B_6 deficiencies.[16] Vitamin B_6 is also thought to improve verbal memory and combat depression.

Vitamin B_9, better known as folic acid, or folate, is critical for brain health. Studies seem to indicate that up to 38 percent of adults who have been clinically diagnosed with depression are deficient in folic acid.[17] Additional research from the Universities of Oxford (England) and Bergen (Norway) report that low folate and low vitamin B_{12} levels are connected to an increased risk of developing Alzheimer's disease. Both studies concluded that the risk for eventually getting Alzheimer's can be dramatically reduced by supplementation with folate and vitamin B_{12}.[18]

I recommend you take a vitamin B complex that provides the daily amounts of all B vitamins as listed on the chart that follows.

VITAMIN C A powerful antioxidant, vitamin C protects against inflammation within our bodies, working to protect our brains against the effects of poor blood flow associated with atherosclerosis. Because vitamin C is water-soluble and rapidly excreted from the body, it is important that levels be replenished daily. I recommend you take 1–3 grams daily.

VITAMIN E Vitamin E (tocopherol) is an antioxidant that helps protect tissue from unhealthy oxidative free radicals, which can cause damage and lead to premature aging and the development of chronic diseases, such as cancer, Alzheimer's, and cataract formation. There are a number of forms of vitamin E. The most common vitamin E supplement is alpha-tocopherol. Recent studies, however, suggest that gamma-tocopherol is the most effective form of vitamin E.

When choosing a vitamin E supplement, look for one containing compounds called tocotrienols, which synergistically combine with vitamin E to help protect our bodies against damaging processes. Tocotrienols also lower the levels of LDL (the dangerous form of cholesterol), which is an important risk factor for heart attack and stroke (remember, this directly affects the brain).

I suggest you choose a vitamin E supplement that has 400 IU of alpha-tocopherol, 200 mg of gamma-tocopherol, and 65 mg of tocotrienols.

SELENIUM This vital mineral can be found in grains, garlic, meat, seafood (oysters, swordfish, tuna), and Brazil nuts. It is a powerful antioxidant that may protect against heart attack and stroke. Selenium appears to encourage a healthy cardiovascular system by increasing the ratio of good cholesterol (HDL) to bad cholesterol (LDL). A healthy cardiovascular system means a healthy flow of nutrient-rich blood to the brain. To promote brain health, I recommend taking 200 mcg of selenium daily.

"Smart" Drugs and Nutrients

A revolution of sorts occurred in the 1970s, when reports began to surface that specific nutrients and drugs could improve concentration, learning, and memory in general, and overall cognitive functions. Choline, phosphatidylcholine, ginkgo biloba, dimethylaminoethanol (DMAE), and phosphatidylserine were the nutrients heading the list. In the drug category, hydergine, piracetam, and centrophenoxine were at the forefront.

ACETYL-L-CARNITINE (ACL) A form of the amino acid–like compound carnitine, acetyl-L-carnitine, or ACL, is produced naturally in the brain. Carnitine transports fatty acids to cells for conversion into energy used by the body's muscles, organs, and tissues. Carnitine deficiencies can place a strain on the heart muscles and create an energy drain on the body that may leave you feeling worn out. A simple urine test can determine if you have a carnitine deficiency.

Some studies show that acetyl-L-carnitine may boost memory and offer some protection against Alzheimer's disease, especially when taken in combination with alpha-lipoic acid.[19] I recommend a supplement of 2,000 mg daily in two divided doses.

ALPHA-LIPOIC ACID This potent antioxidant dissolves in both water and fat, and is thus able to scavenge damaging free radicals more effectively than most antioxidants, which dissolve in either water or fat, but not both. Because it dissolves in fat, alpha-lipoic acid can reach tissues in the nervous system. Results from animal studies show that alpha-lipoic acid may improve long-term memory and holds promise for protection against Alzheimer's disease, particularly when taken in combination with acetyl-L-carnitine.[20] I recommend taking a supplement of 300 mg daily in two divided doses.

CARNOSINE This amino acid compound protects against damage by free radicals and is highly concentrated in the brain. Levels of this powerful antioxidant decline in the body as we age, and supplementing with carnosine may offer benefits in protecting against neurological degeneration. I recommend supplementing with 1,000 mg daily.

COENZYME Q10 (COQ10) As we age, our body's natural production of coenzyme Q10 (coQ10) diminishes. Our older bodies produce only 50 percent of the coQ10 they did when we were younger. This makes coQ10 one of the most important nutrients for people over thirty. Because the cells of our body need coQ10 to produce energy and to combat mitochondrial free radical activity, a coQ10 deficiency can result in a greater incidence of many degenerative diseases associated with aging.

Though the heart is frequently affected by a coQ10 deficiency, scientific reports show that the brain is also likely to suffer adversely from an inadequate supply of coQ10.[21]

CoQ10 is a fat-soluble nutrient that goes into the mitochondria throughout the body. Once there, it governs the oxidation of fats and sugars into energy. When consumed in an oil-based capsule, the coQ10 can be absorbed through the lymphatic canals for better distribution throughout the entire body.

I recommend taking a supplement of 100–300 mg daily with meals for general brain health.

DHEA Youthful hormone balance is vital in maintaining health and preventing disease in individuals over the age of forty. One hormone that is deficient in virtually everyone who is over thirty-five is DHEA (dehydroepiandrosterone).

A large body of research indicates that DHEA is a critically important hormone that appears to protect the entire body against the ravages of aging. Studies on rats have shown that DHEA increases acetylcholine release in the hippocampus of the brain[22] and has improved both short- and long-term memory in mice.[23] Still another study shows that DHEA can protect against early changes in the brain cells associated with Alzheimer's disease.[24]

Not everyone, however, can take advantage of the multiple benefits of DHEA. Men and women with hormone-related cancers, for example, should not take DHEA. This supplement is only available by prescription from your doctor. But if your doctor says it's safe for you, I recommend taking a supplement of 25–50 mg daily.

DMAE This nutrient, found in sardines, is a powerful brain stimulant that increases acetylcholine levels. Acetylcholine is a neurotransmitter associated with mood and energy levels. I recommend taking a supplement of 150 mg daily.

GLYCERYLPHOSPHORYLCHOLINE (GPC) Choline and lecithin can reduce arterial plaque and lower blood pressure. They also enhance acetylcholine production, which plays an important role in memory and learning. One type of choline, called glycerylphosphorylcholine

(GPC), has been shown to improve the condition of subjects with adult-onset cognitive dysfunction, Alzheimer's disease, and stroke-related mental impairment. The therapeutic effects of GPC were noted as superior to either choline or lecithin alone. I recommend a dosage of 600 mg of GPC and 1 gram of lecithin daily.

HYDERGINE Initially discovered in the 1940s, this drug was approved by the FDA for treatment of symptoms of dementia. Today it is used proactively, to protect us against mental decline. Studies support my contention that hydergine protects the brain against age-related decline by enhancing glucose use,[25] increases intelligence, memory, learning, and recall,[26] and increases the blood and oxygen supply to the brain, enhancing metabolism in brain cells.[27] I recommend a daily supplement of 5–10 mg.

PHOSPHATIDYLCHOLINE Phosphatidylcholine is a phospholipid, a large molecule that covers the nerve cells that assist in transferring information between cells. A lack of phospholipids can result in abnormal brain activity and difficulties in the central nervous system. I recommend a supplement of 500–1,000 mg daily.

PS (PHOSPHATIDYLSERINE) PS helps the brain use fuel more efficiently. By boosting neuronal metabolism and stimulating production of acetylcholine, PS may be able to improve the condition of patients in cognitive decline. Studies have revealed that supplementing with phosphatidylserine slows down—and even reverses—declining memory and concentration, or age-related cognitive impairment in middle-aged and elderly subjects.[28] An added benefit is its ability to reduce levels of the stress hormone cortisol.

Phosphatidylserine is a phospholipid that is found in all cells, but is most highly concentrated in the walls (membranes) of brain cells, making up about 70 percent of its nerve tissue mass. There it aids in the storage, release, and activity of many vital neurotransmitters and their receptors. Phosphatidylserine also aids in cell-to-cell communication. It also stimulates the release of dopamine (a mood regulator that also controls physical sensations and movement), increases the production of acetylcholine (necessary for learning and memory), enhances brain glucose metabolism (the fuel used for brain activity), reduces cortisol levels (a stress hormone), and boosts the activity of nerve growth factor (NGF), which oversees the health of cholinergic neurons.

As we grow older, aging slows the body's manufacturing of phosphatidylserine to levels that are detrimental to our functioning at our full mental capacity. This is where supplementation with phosphatidylserine comes into play. In one Belgian study that looked at the effects of phosphatidylserine, thirty-five senile demented patients, aged sixty-five to ninety-one, were hospitalized with mild to moderate memory problems. Seventeen patients were given, over the period of six weeks, phosphatidylserine at 300 milligrams per day. The other eighteen patients received a placebo. The study reported an improved quality of life for the patients who were given phosphatidylserine. Using three different evaluation methods, the researchers classified forty-nine functions—for example, getting dressed, eating, control of bowel and bladder movements—into ten categories. The results were astonishing, as improvements in all ten categories were reported.[29]

I recommend taking a supplement of 300 mg daily.

PREGNENOLONE A hormone produced by the adrenal glands, pregnenolone is abundant in the brain, where it facilitates communication between neurotransmitters. As we age, the amount of pregnenolone our bodies produce declines; levels can be tested by a basic urine test. I recommend a daily supplement of 50 mg pregnenolone.

PROANTHOCYANIDINS Proanthocyanidins (chemical relatives of bioflavonoids) serve to benefit the brain in a twofold manner: they are antioxidants and they protect collagen.

Brace yourself for what I am about to tell you. Research has shown that proanthocyanidins are fifty times more powerful antioxidants than vitamins C and E! Intricate tests prove that proanthocyanidins are great killers of the hydroxyl radical—the free radical that is responsible for the most damage—and lipid peroxides (rancid fats).[30] This is extremely important because the brain is particularly vulnerable to free radical damage.

In protecting collagen, proanthocyanidins are, in essence, protecting the glue that holds the brain together. Enzymes can destroy the wall of blood vessels that is, essentially, collagen. Proanthocyanidins therefore protect the blood-brain barrier. Remember, the blood-brain barrier protects the brain

from toxins and other potentially destructive substances. Thus, proanthocyanidins, as potent shields of the blood-brain barrier, are invaluable.

Although proanthocyanidins can be found in the diet, the levels in
food are generally insufficient to provide the brain with the fortification it
needs to ward off attack. Thus, the best way to obtain proanthocyanidins is
through supplementation. In particular, the best two sources are grape seed
extract and pine bark extract. I recommend supplementing with 80 mg
daily.

TMG (TRIMETHYLGLYCINE) TMG is the most effective facil-
itator of youthful methylation metabolism. Research has shown that defective methylation is implicated in a variety of diseases, including cancer,
neurological disorders, and birth defects.[31] Methylation produces SAMe
(S-adenosylmethionine), which may have powerful anti-aging effects and
has eased depression and improved Parkinson's symptoms in patients with
the disease. TMG should be taken with vitamin B_6 and folic acid to enhance
the effectiveness of methylation. I recommend taking 200–300 mg per day.

VINPOCETINE Vinpocetine is an extract taken from the lesser periwinkle plant (*vinca minor*). It is available by prescription in Europe and is
used for boosting stroke- and age-related decline in brain function. In the
United States, it is available as an over-the-counter dietary supplement.
Vinpocetine may provide protection against the types of cognitive decline
associated with poor brain circulation, including memory loss and disorientation. It also enhances the brain's use of oxygen by boosting levels of
adenosine triphosphate (ATP), an important brain fuel. I recommend a
dose of 10 mg twice daily with meals.

Mind Power Chart of Daily Supplements for Best Brain Health

Supplemental vitamins and minerals, as well as smart nutrients and drugs,
can be extremely beneficial to our brain health when used in combination
with a healthful diet. But I know keeping track of the proper dosages can be
difficult. To help you in that goal, I have provided the following chart that
summarizes the supplement program I recommend.

The plan that follows is intended to promote brain health and protect
your brain. In Part 2 of this book, I discuss specific conditions and recommend vitamins and supplements that can be added to this basic plan to fight

and impact brain conditions like memory loss, Parkinson's disease, or headaches. When recommending protocols for specific conditions, I am assuming that you are already following the supplement program in the chart that follows.

Do not combine this protocol with more than one additional protocol from Part 2 of this book. If you are taking medications, or have any food restrictions, you should consult with your doctor before beginning this or any supplement program. Supplement overdoses are rare, but possible, and certain combinations may affect individuals adversely.

Vitamins and Nutrients	Daily Dose	Comments
acetyl–L–carnitine (ACL)	2,000 mg in two divided doses	
alpha–lipoic acid	300 mg in two divided doses	
B-complex vitamins	<ul><li>100 mg thiamine (B_1)</li><li>50 mg riboflavin (B_2)</li><li>200 mg niacin (B_3)</li><li>1,000 mg pantothenic acid (B_5)</li><li>75 mg pyridoxine (B_6)</li><li>250 mg inositol (B_8)</li><li>800 mcg folic acid (B_9)</li><li>100 mcg vitamin B_{12}</li><li>60 mcg biotin</li><li>200–300 mg trimethylglycine (TMG)</li><li>45 mg choline</li><li>100 mg para-aminobenzoic acid</li></ul>	A B-complex vitamin should contain the dosages I recommend.
carnosine	1,000 mg	
coenzyme Q10 (coQ10)	100–300 mg with meals	
dehydroepiandrosterone (DHEA)	25–50 mg	Must be prescribed by health practitioner. Individuals with hormone-related

Vitamins and Nutrients	Daily Dose	Comments
dehydroepiandrosterone (DHEA) (*cont.*)		cancers should not take DHEA.
dimethylaminoethanol (DMAE)	150 mg	May be overstimulating for some people. Headaches, muscle tension, and irritability may occur. Do not take if you have epilepsy, a history of convulsions, or bipolar disorder. If you have kidney or liver disease, consult your doctor before taking this supplement.
essential fatty acids (EFAs)	• 4,000 mg borage oil (equals 920 mg GLA) • 2,000 mg fish oil extract (equals 1,000 mg DHA) • 400 mg EFP	
glycerylphosphorylcholine (GPC)	600 mg	
hydergine	5–10 mg	
lecithin	1 gram	About 1 heaping tablespoon of granules
phosphatidylcholine	500–1,000 mg	
phosphatidylserine (PS)	300 mg	Do not use if you have a bipolar disorder; do not use if you suffer from depression.
pregnenolone	50 mg	Individuals with hormone-related

continued...

Vitamins and Nutrients	Daily Dose	Comments
pregnenolone (*cont.*)		cancers should not take pregnenolone.
proanthocyanidins	80 mg	Naturally occurring in grape seed extract and pine bark extract.
selenium	200 mcg	
vinpocetine	10 mg two times daily with meals	
vitamin C	1–3 grams	
vitamin E	400 IU 200 mg (gamma-tocopherol) 65 mg (palm oil–derived tocotrienols)	Mixed tocopherols with an emphasis on gamma

SUMMARY

In this chapter I have shown you a plan for protecting brain health, no matter what your age. By following these nutritional guidelines and supplementing with essential vitamins, minerals, and smart drugs, you are taking an important step in safeguarding your brain against age-related decline. These measures are for all of us. They are preventive at the very least.

In the chapters that follow in Part 2, I address specific conditions that affect our brains and mental health. I offer a detailed protocol of diet, nutrition, supplements, and alternative therapies that can rejuvenate your brain and eliminate many of the symptoms and diseases that are associated with age-related mental decline. These individualized protocols should be followed *in addition to* the basic Mind Power plan in this chapter.

PART II

SPECIFIC BRAIN CONDITIONS
AND TREATMENTS

AN IMPORTANT NOTE ABOUT SUPPLEMENTS AND MULTIPLE CONDITIONS

This book is designed for individuals who have, or are specifically concerned about, only one of the conditions discussed in the following chapters. To promote brain health and protect your brain, you should follow my protocol for optimal brain health in Chapter 2.

In the chapters in this section, I'll recommend protocols for specific brain conditions. The vitamins, minerals, and supplements I recommend should be incorporated into the protocol from Chapter 2. In some cases I will recommend increasing the dose of a particular vitamin or supplement to impact a specific condition. In these cases, you should increase the daily dosage from Chapter 2 to the level recommended for that specific condition.

Do not combine the protocols in these chapters with each other. And do not add more than one additional protocol to the one given in Chapter 2. If you are concerned about more than one of the brain conditions discussed in this section, consult with a health professional about how you can safely impact multiple conditions. If you are taking medications, or have any food restrictions, you should consult with your doctor before beginning any supplement program. Supplement overdoses are rare, but possible, and certain combinations may affect individuals adversely.

CHAPTER 3

DEPRESSION

The perceived link between aging and depression has been a real concern of mine for most of my career. As far as I'm concerned, the notion that suffering depression is an inherent risk of the aging process is absolutely false: depression is absolutely *not* a by-product of aging. In my experience, many older people feel satisfied with their lives; they are vital, fulfilled, energetic individuals. It would not be considered normal for them to suffer from depression. In fact, there is nothing "normal" about depression at any age, and there is certainly no need to tolerate it simply because we are growing older.

Of course, anyone can feel sad or "down" at times, but these moods should pass. When these blue periods impact behavior, thinking, emotion, memory, energy levels, or physical health over an extended period of time, then a diagnosis of clinical depression must be considered. Unfortunately the incidence of diagnosed depression is increasing in the aging population. Late-life depression affects about 6 million Americans age sixty-five and older. The National Institutes of Health has named late-life depression as a major public health problem.[1]

Depression is manifested both physically and emotionally. It affects the whole person—body, mind, and spirit. Any steps to overcome it must address all of these areas. Depression is difficult to self-diagnose, and often, equally difficult for medical professionals to pinpoint.

In this chapter, I'll start by discussing the different types of depression and their causes. Then I'll give you some guidelines for determining if you are suffering from depression. Once you know where you stand, I'll discuss the lifestyle and nutritional strategies you can use to fight depression naturally.

UNDERSTANDING DEPRESSION

Your brain uses neurotransmitters to send information between nerve cells. When the neurotransmitter levels are low, messages cannot flow smoothly across the synaptic gaps. In essence, the communication in your brain becomes sluggish. When the delicate balance of these compounds is disrupted, depression may occur.

There are three main neurotransmitters directly related to depression:

Serotonin: Individuals with low serotonin levels are likely to be depressed or experience internal anger. When the brain creates serotonin, tension is eased.

Dopamine: An intermediate in the synthesis of epinephrine, dopamine is a compound that prepares the body to meet emergencies such as cold, fatigue, or shock. Low levels can affect sleep, appetite, mood, and sexual interest.

Norepinephrine: Related to the chemical epinephrine, norepinephrine is released in response to short-term stress. An excess release of norepinephrine can cause increased heart rate and blood pressure, an increase in glycogenolysis (the conversion of glycogen to glucose), and an increase in lipolysis (the conversion of fats to fatty acids) in fat tissues. Like dopamine, increased norepinephrine levels can have a positive effect on some of the symptoms of depression.

Let's start with a look at the different types of depression and how you can tell if you are suffering from one of them.

Types of Depression

The cause of depression can generally be attributed to one of three broad categories: life events, a chemical imbalance induced by certain medications or environmental factors, or genetics and family history.

Dysthymia

Dysthymia is the most common type of depressive disorder. This type of *reactive* depression can occur at any time, triggered by an agonizing or anxiety-producing event. When afflicted with this disorder, an individual can function at a basic level, but may lose interest in formerly pleasurable activities.

Clinical Depression

Clinical depression is not related to an external event, but is brought on by an imbalance of chemicals in the brain. There are strong indications this may be a result of an individual having a genetic predisposition for this condition. More severe than reactive depression, clinical depression may cause an individual to experience an *extreme* loss of interest in practically everything. And, unlike reactive depression, it has the potential to adversely affect all aspects of everyday living.

Manic Depression

Manic depression is characterized by severe mood swings. A person with manic depression will fluctuate between periods of extreme energy and vivacity and those of complete hopelessness. The causes of manic depression are not fully known, although there are inherited components.[2] Chemical imbalances in the brain may play a role, and stressful or traumatic events may provide the trigger for an episode of mania or depression.

Contagious Depression

Some researchers also believe that depression is contagious. Dr. Ronald M. Podell, in his book *Contagious Emotions: Staying Well When Your Loved One Is Depressed,*[3] reports that when a spouse is continually depressed, the other spouse will eventually become depressed as well.

Heavy Metal Contamination

Dr. Lewis Harrison posits that depression may result from heavy metal contamination of the body.[4] Aluminum, lead, copper, and mercury are present in our cooking utensils, the wiring in our homes, our drinking water, the fish we eat, even in the dental fillings in our teeth. Removing these metals from our bodies through a thorough detoxification program can be beneficial in preventing and impacting depression. To learn more about detoxification programs, visit my Web site: www.garynull.com.

Parasite Poisoning

Dr. Hazel Parcells has done extensive work on the connection between depression and parasitic infection. Natural remedies such as garlic, pumpkin seeds, grapefruit seed extract, and olive leaf extract have been found to be effective against a range of parasitic invaders.[5]

Diagnosing Depression

Many physicians today are inclined to use depression as a catchall diagnosis for an array of symptoms that can't be traced to a physical cause. Below, I list the most common symptoms of depression as they are manifested in older people. Anyone experiencing these symptoms every day for more than two weeks should be evaluated by a health professional to see if they are suffering from depression.

Symptoms of Depression

The common symptoms of depression include a long list of behaviors:

- agitation
- anxiety
- persistent, vague physical complaints
- difficulty concentrating or remembering things
- lack of interest in social activities
- loss of appetite
- unexplained weight loss or weight gain
- sleep disturbances such as insomnia, oversleeping, or early-morning waking
- irritability or overly demanding behavior
- lack of attention to personal care or hygiene
- confusion or delusion
- feelings of hopelessness
- sadness, excessive crying
- loss of interest in normally pleasurable activities, such as sex
- loss of self-worth
- prolonged grief after a loss
- low energy, fatigue, feeling of "slowing down"
- suicidal thoughts

As we age, we all experience an accumulation of negative life events. We may suffer from serious or chronic physical illnesses or impaired functioning. What makes age-related depression difficult to diagnose is that it shares symptoms with many other conditions, including Parkinson's, Alzheimer's, dementia, thyroid disorders, strokes, heart disease, and side effects of medications. Sleep disturbances, weight loss, and low energy can be symptoms of diabetes or heart disease. Poor concentration, apathy, and memory loss are found in Parkinson's and Alzheimer's diseases. Fatigue may be a side effect of certain medications. And general aches and pains may result from a lack of—or overexertion in—activity or exercise. These common experiences of aging make the diagnosis of depression especially difficult for the elderly.

Geriatric Depression Scale

Because of the difficulties in obtaining a diagnosis of depression in older adults, the Geriatric Depression Scale (GDS)[6] was developed to gauge depression specifically in the elderly. This series of thirty questions can provide an indicator of whether an older person is suffering from depression.

Circle the answer that best represents how you felt this week:

1. Are you basically satisfied with your life?   yes   no
2. Have you dropped many of your activities
    and interests?   yes   no
3. Do you feel that your life is empty?   yes   no
4. Do you often get bored?   yes   no
5. Are you hopeful about the future?   yes   no
6. Are you bothered by thoughts you can't dismiss? yes   no
7. Are you in good spirits most of the time?   yes   no
8. Are you afraid something bad is going to
    happen to you?   yes   no
9. Do you feel happy most of the time?   yes   no
10. Do you often feel helpless?   yes   no
11. Do you often get restless and fidgety?   yes   no
12. Do you prefer to stay home rather than go out
    and do things?   yes   no
13. Do you frequently worry about the future?   yes   no
14. Do you feel you have more problems with
    memory than most?   yes   no
15. Do you think it is wonderful to be alive now?   yes   no
16. Do you often feel downhearted and blue?   yes   no
17. Do you feel pretty worthless the way you are now? yes   no
18. Do you worry a lot about the past?   yes   no
19. Do you find life very exciting?   yes   no

20.	Is it hard for you to get started on new projects?	yes	no
21.	Do you feel full of energy?	yes	no
22.	Do you feel that your situation is hopeless?	yes	no
23.	Do you think that most people are better off than you are?	yes	no
24.	Do you frequently get upset over little things?	yes	no
25.	Do you frequently feel like crying?	yes	no
26.	Do you have trouble concentrating?	yes	no
27.	Do you enjoy getting up in the morning?	yes	no
28.	Do you avoid social gatherings?	yes .	no
29.	Is it easy for you to make decisions?	yes	no
30.	Is your mind as clear as it used to be?	yes	no

Scoring Your Test

Calculate your score accordingly:

Give yourself 1 point for every "yes" answer to questions 2, 3, 4, 6, 8, 10, 11, 12, 13, 14, 16, 18, 20, 22, 23, 24, 25, 26, and 28.

Give yourself 1 point for every "no" answer to questions 1, 5, 7, 9, 15, 19, 21, 27, 29, and 30.

Total your points.

0–9 points = normal

10–19 points = mildly depressed

20–30 points = very depressed

COMBATING DEPRESSION NATURALLY

Now, if you were to take this test and become concerned about the state of your mental health, you might go to your doctor. You might complain about sleeping problems, low energy, poor concentration and memory loss, or even general aches and fatigue. And it is likely that your doctor will conclude you are suffering from depression. But rather than examining other factors, such as nutritional or hormone deficiencies that may be contributing to your depression, your doctor will probably suggest you begin taking antidepressant medication as a course of treatment.

What you must keep in mind is that while drug therapy with antidepressants, such as Prozac, can help people feel better, there are negative side effects to these drugs and we do not know what the long-term effects are. What we do know is that, in general, depression must be viewed as a mind *and* body disorder, and that the relationship between depression and environmental and physical factors is a complex one. Everyone's situation and needs are unique.

In the Mind Power protocol for impacting depression that follows, I recommend natural approaches that treat the body and mind gently. I will teach you not only how to impact the symptoms of depression, but perhaps more important, how to focus on overcoming the fundamental causes of the condition. You will learn how to use nutrition, supplements, and lifestyle changes to *naturally* prevent and control the symptoms of depression and to rejuvenate and protect your long-term physical and mental health.

Lifestyle

Life events and anxiety-provoking situations can trigger depression. By consciously making lifestyle choices that promote physical, mental, and emotional health, we create a mind/body balance that allows us to access vital tools for preventing and reversing depression.

Exercise

Exercise is an important factor in preventing depression, and equally important in overcoming the condition. The lasting effect of regular exercise is an increased energy level and a feeling of revitalization and accomplishment. Even the most moderate and mild type of exercise can be beneficial.

When you are depressed, your energy levels are low and it can be hard to start any kind of activity. Begin with simple movements, such as going for a walk, or performing stretches while seated. Active hobbies, such as gardening or dancing, are pleasurable ways to introduce increased exercise into your life.

As you move more, you will experience a positive effect on both your mind and your body, and it will become easier to include exercise as a regular part of your daily activities.

Social Interactions

The nature of depression can interfere with a person's ability to seek assistance. Depression saps energy and self-esteem. Positive social encounters can make the difference between suffering and recovery.

Spending time with friends and family of all ages is important in remaining vital and connected. Emotional support can help us to weather a crisis of loss or grief. Humor lifts our moods and opens us to experiencing daily happiness. Volunteering to help others, learning new skills, and participating in absorbing and pleasurable activities enhance feelings of worth at any age. Spiritual communities may offer comfort and promote positive feelings. Loving touch is a proven mood elevator: massage, hugs—even stroking a pet—can lift our mood.

Environment

Music, visual and dramatic arts, even color can affect mood. There are therapists who specialize in using creative expression to help with mental health issues. Music, dance, and journaling help some individuals understand and process complex emotions. Our physical environment is a reflection of our emotional, spiritual, and intellectual state. Adjusting the elements in our environment can have a miraculous effect in fighting and overcoming depression.

Nutrition

What can be difficult in promoting proper nutrition as we age is the fact that our bodies may become less efficient in absorbing and utilizing key nutrients. Furthermore, someone suffering from depression may have little or no appetite or interest in food. Therefore, it is important that every bit of food you eat has the maximum positive impact on your mental health.

Foods and Depression

The first step in eating a brain-healthy diet is to eliminate fast foods, simple carbohydrates, alcohol, artificial sweeteners, white flour products, and caffeine. This change will immediately improve the chemical balances in your brain.

To prevent and combat depression, your diet should contain lots of fruits and vegetables, with soybeans and soy products, brown rice, millet and legumes and essential fatty acids. Placebo-controlled research conducted with medicated patients suggests that adding omega-3 fatty acids, particularly eicosapentaenoic acid, may ameliorate symptoms of major depressive disorder.[7]

At all costs, you must avoid meat or fried foods, such as hamburgers and french fries. These foods are high in saturated fats that block the arteries and small blood vessels, interfering with blood flow. Your blood cells become sticky and clump together, leading to poor cerebral circulation, accompanied by mental sluggishness and fatigue.

Depressed people are attracted to sugar because of the initial lift it provides. Sugar does stimulate serotonin levels, which in turn temporarily improves your mood. But this initial surge of energy disappears in a matter of minutes. The reason behind the initial boost is that sugar—regardless of which form you are talking about—does not have to be digested and passes directly into the bloodstream, where it dramatically raises the blood sugar level, and overstimulates the pancreas to produce too much insulin. The excess insulin then causes the sugar level to plummet. Within half an hour of consuming a sugary snack, your blood sugar level will drop to very low levels, allowing fatigue, irritability, and anxiety to creep in. With these feelings present, the person seeks another boost from sugar, resulting in repeating the same, vicious cycle.

Recipes

The recipes at the end of this book are intended to help you get started on a healthy eating plan that will provide optimum mental health benefits. Each dish focuses on foods rich in vitamins and nutrients beneficial to our brains. Eating right does not have to involve a huge effort. Prepare healthy dishes in larger quantities and store them for use throughout the week. In the list below are my recommendations for easy-to-prepare meals full of nutrients proven to help prevent depression.

Pasta Fagioli, page 288
Sweet Kidney Bean Mash, page 290
Heavenly Roasted Nuts, page 296

Supplements

Even with a diet rich in recommended vitamins and minerals, your body may not efficiently absorb and process these necessary nutrients. As you grow older, your appetite may decrease, and you may find that you are unable to consistently take in the recommended amounts of food nutrients. Furthermore, loss of appetite is a common symptom of depression. It may be that getting these nutrients in supplement form is the most efficient way for you to enhance your healthy diet. However, supplements are not intended to replace healthy food choices.

Of course, before you begin any new health program, you should get a comprehensive, full-body evaluation performed by a qualified health care practitioner. A proper health and medical evaluation should evaluate your blood chemistry to assess your blood markers, your metabolic rate, and your blood pressure for indicators of cardiovascular, hormonal, or other imbalances or danger signs. If you are taking medications of any sort, for depression or any other condition, you need to inform your doctor of any supplements you are considering adding to your daily diet, as some may interact with prescription medications and cause adverse effects. You should speak to your doctor before adding any of these supplements to your daily regimen.

Vitamins and Minerals

Certain vitamins and minerals are especially important in fighting depression.

FOLIC ACID Folic acid levels are directly related to the severity of depression: the lower the level of folic acid in the blood, the more serious the level of depression. Low levels of folic acid have been linked to depression and bipolar disorder in a number of studies. Insufficient folic acid is one of the most common nutritional deficiencies, and one-third of all adults are low in this important vitamin.[8] I recommend that your daily B-complex vitamin contain at least 800 mcg of folic acid. If you are taking folic acid as a separate supplement, always combine it with 1,000 mcg of vitamin B_{12}.

VITAMIN B$_{12}$ Vitamin B$_{12}$ deficiency may also play a part in depression. As we age, it becomes increasingly difficult for our bodies to absorb sufficient amounts of B$_{12}$ from what we eat. So even if you are consuming *adequate* quantities of foods rich in B$_{12}$, your body is not getting the full benefit. I recommend that your daily B-complex vitamin contain at least 1,000 mcg of vitamin B$_{12}$.

VITAMIN B$_6$ Vitamin B$_6$ converts tryptophan (an amino acid) into serotonin. While extreme deficiencies in B$_6$ are rare, minor deficiencies— which occur frequently—can lead to depression. Heavy users of alcohol are likely to have a B$_6$ deficiency, as are women who use oral contraceptives. I recommend that your daily B-complex vitamin contain at least 75 mg of vitamin B$_6$.

VITAMIN D Vitamin D is called the sunlight vitamin because the body produces it when the sun's ultraviolet B (UVB) rays strike the skin. It is the only vitamin the body manufactures naturally. Considered a mood elevator, vitamin D may be effective in dealing with seasonal depression. Ten to fifteen minutes of summer sun a few days per week generally supplies the body with sufficient amounts of vitamin D. Our body's ability to produce vitamin D declines as we age, however, and those who are unable to spend time outside, or who suffer the effects of the lack of sun in winter climates, may want to supplement. For those suffering from depression, I recommend supplementing with 400–600 IU of vitamin D daily.

INOSITOL Inositol—also known as B$_8$—functions closely with lecithin and choline. It is a fundamental ingredient of cell membranes and is necessary for proper brain function. The neurotransmitter serotonin depends upon inositol to function properly. I recommend increasing your daily inositol supplement from 250 mg to 2,250 mg. Do not exceed 2,250 mg daily.

MAGNESIUM Magnesium deficiency is also seen in people suffering from depression. When patients recover from depression, magnesium levels in the blood rise.[9] Magnesium supplements should be taken with calcium to lessen overreaction to stress and panic attacks. I recommend that women suffering from depression take a supplement of 320 mg daily; men should take a supplement of 420 mg daily.

POTASSIUM Potassium is one of the most abundant minerals in the human body. Most of the time supplementation with potassium is unnecessary, because it is so readily available in our diet in such foods as bananas, orange juice, and potatoes. Potassium is depleted from our bodies in times of stress, thus upsetting the delicate balance of neurotransmitter communication in our brains. For this reason, potassium supplements may be useful in impacting depression. Potassium can interact with some drugs, so if you are taking prescription medications, consult with your doctor before taking potassium supplements. If potassium is safe for you, I recommend a daily supplement of 500 mg.

Smart Drugs and Nutrients

A number of other naturally occurring nutrients may have beneficial impacts on depression.

5-HTP (5-HYDROXYTRYPTOPHAN) A derivative of the amino acid tryptophan, this mood-enhancing chemical is converted into the neurotransmitter serotonin. 5-HTP should be taken with carbidopa, a decarboxylase inhibitor that prevents 5-HTP from converting to serotonin before it reaches the brain. For depression, anxiety, and panic attacks, I recommend taking 50–100 mg three times daily.

ADAPTON (GARUM ARMORICUM) This naturally occurring substance is taken from a deep-sea fish. It is widely used in Europe and Japan to help with stress, anxiety, and depression. It improves concentration, mood, and sleep. You should take 4 capsules as directed for fifteen days; stop for one week, then continue with a maintenance dose of 2 capsules daily.

DHEA Youthful hormone balance is vital in maintaining health and preventing disease in individuals over the age of forty. One hormone that is deficient in virtually everyone who is over thirty-five is DHEA (dehydroepiandrosterone). This building block for estrogen and testosterone enhances mood and a sense of well-being in menopausal women.

Not everyone, however, can take advantage of the multiple benefits of DHEA. Men and women with hormone-related cancers, for example, should not take DHEA. This supplement is only available by prescription from your doctor. If your doctor says it's safe for you, I recommend taking a supplement of 25–50 mg daily; if your doctor thinks DHEA will help in the treatment of your depression, they will prescribe an appropriate increase in your dosage.

DLPA (DL-PHENYLALANINE) DLPA contains two forms ("D" and "L") of the amino acid phenylalanine. The "L" form is naturally occurring and believed to bolster mood-elevating chemicals in the brain. The "D" form is a synthetic form of a substance that has a pain-relieving effect. In one clinical trial of individuals suffering from depression, twelve of twenty depressed men and women who took 75–200 mg of DLPA daily reported being free of depression after nearly three weeks of treatment, and four reported feeling somewhat better.[10]

You should not combine DLPA with prescription antidepressants or stimulants unless specifically directed to do so by your doctor. If you have high blood pressure, or are prone to panic attacks, DLPA may aggravate your condition. DLPA should also not be used if you are taking levodopa for treatment of Parkinson's disease. Women who are pregnant, or individuals with melanoma, should not take DLPA. People with PKU (a rare, inherited metabolism disorder) should avoid DLPA as well.

If you are able to take DLPA, I recommend a supplement of 1,000–1,500 mg daily.

DMAE (DIMETHYLAMINOETHANOL) This nutrient, found in sardines, is a powerful brain stimulant that increases acetylcholine levels. Acetylcholine is a neurotransmitter associated with mood and energy levels. I recommend increasing your daily supplement from 150 mg to 650–1,650 mg daily. Do not exceed 1,650 mg daily.

PREGNENOLONE A hormone produced by the adrenal glands, pregnenolone is abundant in the brain, where it facilitates communication between neurotransmitters. Low levels of pregnenolone have been linked to depression. As we age, the amount of pregnenolone we produce declines; levels can be tested by a basic urine test. To improve your ability to handle the stress brought on by depression, I recommend increasing your daily supplement from 50 mg to 100–250 mg daily. Do not exceed 250 mg daily.

SAME (S-ADENOSYLMETHIONINE) SAMe (pronounced "sammy") has long been prescribed by European doctors as a treatment for depression. SAMe promotes cell growth and repair, and maintains levels of glutathione, a major antioxidant that protects against free radicals and contributes to the formation of the mood-enhancing neurotransmitter serotonin. SAMe should not be taken if you are taking MAO inhibitor antidepressants. You should consult with your doctor before taking SAMe if you suffer from severe depression or bipolar disorder. If SAMe is safe for you to use, I recommend a supplement of 400–800 mg taken twice daily.

Mind Power Chart of Additional Supplements for Impacting Depression

The following chart summarizes the supplements I recommend adding to the protocol for overall brain health from Chapter 2. In some cases I will recommend increasing the dose of a particular vitamin or supplement to specifically impact depression. In these cases, you should increase the daily dosage from Chapter 2 to the level recommended for that specific condition.

This protocol is designed for individuals who suffer from, or are specifically concerned about, depression. If you are concerned about additional brain conditions discussed in other chapters, consult with a health professional about how you can safely impact multiple conditions.

If you are taking medications—whether prescription or over-the-counter—or have any food restrictions, consult with your doctor before beginning any supplement program. Your health care provider should always be up-to-date on all vitamins, supplements, and herbal or homeopathic remedies you are taking. Supplement overdoses are rare, but possible, and certain combinations may affect individuals adversely.

Supplement	Dosage	Cautions
5-HTP (5-hydroxytryptophan)	50–100 mg three times daily	Several months of treatment may be needed for maximum benefit. Nausea is the main side effect, but if it occurs, it usually dissipates within several days. Do not combine with prescription antidepressants.

continued...

Supplement	Dosage	Cautions
5-HTP (5-hydroxytryptophan) (*cont.*)		If you are taking prescription medication for depression, you should consult with your doctor before taking 5-HTP. Excess levels of serotonin in the blood can be dangerous in case of coronary artery disease.
Adapton (*Garum Armoricum*)	4 capsules as directed daily for fifteen days; stop for one week, then continue with maintenance dose of 2 capsules daily.	
DHEA hormone	Follow doctor's directions for dosage.	Must be prescribed by your health practitioner. Individuals with hormone-related cancers should not take DHEA.
DLPA (DL-phenylalanine)	1,000–1,500 mg	Do not combine DLPA with prescription antidepressants or stimulants unless specifically directed to do so by your doctor. Do not take DLPA if you have high blood pressure, or are prone to panic attacks, are taking levodopa for treatment of Parkinson's disease, are pregnant, have melanoma, or have PKU (a rare, inherited metabolism disorder).

Supplement	Dosage	Cautions
DMAE (dimethylaminoethanol)	Increase daily dosage from 150 mg to 650–1,650 mg. Do not exceed a daily supplement of 1,650 mg.	May be overstimulating for some people. Headaches, muscle tension, and irritability may occur. Do not take if you have epilepsy, a history of convulsions, or bipolar disease. If you have kidney or liver disease, consult your doctor before taking this supplement.
inositol	Increase daily dosage from 250 mg to 2,250 mg. Do not exceed a daily supplement of 2,250 mg. Take in two divided doses.	
magnesium	320 mg (for women), 420 mg (for men)	May take six weeks or more for effects to be felt.
potassium	500 mg	Do not take potassium supplements if you are taking medication for high blood pressure or heart disease, or if you have a kidney disorder. Consuming foods rich in potassium is okay. Do not exceed a supplementary dose of 3.5 grams daily without consulting with your doctor.
pregnenolone	Increase daily dosage from 50 mg to 100–250 mg. Do not exceed a daily supplement of 250 mg.	Individuals with hormone-related cancers should not take pregnenolone.

continued...

Supplement	Dosage	Cautions
SAMe (S-adenosylmethionine)	Dosage range of 400–1,600 mg	Raise the dose gradually from 200 mg twice a day to 400 mg twice a day, to 400 mg three times a day, to 400 mg four times a day, over a period of twenty days.
vitamin D	400–600 IU daily	Do not exceed 800 IU daily.

Alternative Health Remedies

When suffering from a specific condition like depression, we can also try some natural treatment options that are considered "alternatives" to traditional medicine. While a healthful lifestyle and the proper nutritional and supplement plan are vital to winning the battle against depression, there are some other targeted remedies that might help, too.

Herbal Remedies

Some herbal extracts and homeopathic treatments have properties similar to conventional medications, but are gentler and may lack the drugs' side effects. Always inform your medical practitioner of any herbal remedies you may be taking.

- **St. John's wort** (*Hypericum*) is very popular in Europe, where double-blind, placebo-controlled studies exist to support its efficacy in alleviating depression.[11] *Hypericum* is taken by more than 20 million people in Germany to combat depression. In fact, it is covered by German health insurance as a prescription drug. I recommend taking 450 mg twice daily.
- **Ginkgo biloba** is an extract of the ginkgo plant, is used in Europe to help fight dementia and Alzheimer's disease, and is a free radical scavenger effective at eliminating free radicals. It increases blood circulation to the brain and protects nerve cells, and has shown promise in impacting mild depression. One study revealed that elderly people

suffering from depression, who showed no improvement on antidepressant drugs, did respond when a ginkgo biloba extract was added.[12] Your daily supplement should be 300 mg in two divided doses.

- **Chinese schisandra berry** is an adaptogen, like ginseng. It redirects energy, calms nerves, and can act as a mild sedative. I recommend taking 100 mg twice daily.
- **Calamus root** can be used externally, by adding it to a bath to induce a state of tranquility. It should be avoided during pregnancy.

Homeopathic Remedies

The following remedies may be used for both temporary and acute cases of depression. When dealing with a chronic condition, homeopathic remedies must be used in conjunction with other therapies, as prescribed by a qualified health professional. Consult with your health care provider before taking any homeopathic remedy, and follow their recommendation for the appropriate dosage. Always inform your medical practitioner of any homeopathic remedies you may be taking.

- **Aurum metallicum** alleviates feelings of worthlessness, low self-esteem, and despair. It can help provide hope for a person with reactive depression, and is said to be particularly beneficial to idealistic and goal-oriented individuals who have experienced life-altering events and feel they have somehow failed.
- **Natrun muriaticum** is used when depression results from an event generating profound bereavement and distress. It is prescribed for people who cannot show their feelings and who suffer in silence, believing they must appear strong and controlled.
- **Sepia** is used mainly for women experiencing depression associated with menopause. This type of depression can be characterized by irritability and indifference to others.
- **Pulsatilla** is used for people who show signs of manic depression.

Light Therapy

In his book *Beyond Prozac*,[13] Dr. Michael Norden states that light therapy has shown positive results in helping patients overcome the mild depression associated with seasonal affective disorder (SAD). The body chemistry of many individuals is thrown off by the decrease in the daylight hours during the winter season. But treatments that utilize bright light have shown promise in overcoming this type of depression. One such treatment is called dawn stimulation, and is a unique lighting system used in the bedroom that is manipulated to mimic sunrise. Using dawn stimulation therapy results in an increased energy level and ease of waking for some individuals.

Light therapy is administered by a 10,000-lux light box, which contains white fluorescent light tubes covered with a plastic screen that blocks ultraviolet rays. An individual sits in front of the box with their eyes open, but not looking directly into the light. Daily sessions of ten to fifteen minutes are gradually increased to thirty- to forty-five-minute sessions. Ninety minutes of exposure per day is often prescribed. This therapy can easily be practiced at home.

Aromatherapy

Essential oils can be used in baths or inhaled to provide rebalancing effects. Do not apply essential oils directly to the skin; they must be mixed with carrier oils. Experiment with various scents to see what you find most soothing or energizing.

- lavender
- basil
- jasmine
- rose
- bergamot
- sandalwood
- neroli (orange blossom oil)
- ylang-ylang
- marjoram
- clary sage
- chamomile

SUMMARY

With careful attention to our diets, our environment, and our physical and spiritual selves, we can enjoy lives rich in vitality, energy, and self-esteem at any age. The Mind Power program works to keep you in balance during stressful or anxious times, allowing you to weather life's experiences without falling victim to debilitating depression.

CHAPTER 4

ANXIETY

Our first day at school, our first date, starting a new job, buying a house, facing a serious illness—many rites of passage are marked by sweaty palms, rapid breathing, and a stomach full of butterflies. Our bodies switch into high gear: we feel alert, ready to react, poised for any possibility. Anxiety is a typical and appropriate reaction to many types of stress. When experienced at an optimum level, anxiety keeps you sharp and allows you to foresee things that need attention.

We experience anxiety throughout our lives; it is part of our genetic makeup. We wouldn't be alive today if our ancestors had lacked the ability to anticipate dangers and threats. A low level of anxiety is as natural a part of our existence as breathing, eating, and sleeping. Dr. Richard Restak, a Clinical Professor of Neurology at George Washington University School of Medicine and Health Sciences in Washington, D.C., describes anxiety as a biological function with a preservative aspect: the ability to use the frontal lobe of our brain to imagine future possibilities. These future possibilities sometimes include events that induce a reaction of anxiety and provoke a particular biochemical reaction in the brain.[1]

When an anxious moment changes from a short-lived period of stimulation to an uncontrollable period of worry and accompanying stress, however, and feelings of restless foreboding become excessive, what is supposed to be a helpful biological reaction becomes a dysfunctional state. Clinical anxiety disorders are marked by an ongoing and pervasive sense of threat and vulnerability. Given our day-to-day living environment—in which we are bombarded by constant news of global terrorism and local crime—it may not surprise you to find out that more than 19 million Americans suffer from some sort of acute anxiety.[2]

Until recently, anxiety disorders were thought to be most prevalent in the younger population. Experts are now beginning to recognize that anxiety disorders are common in the elderly population, however, especially in older people who suffer from depression. In fact, conditions generally associated with aging, such as chronic physical problems, cognitive difficulties, and significant emotional losses, may be triggers for anxiety disorders.

Because anxiety disorders spring from many, often interrelated, causes, the treatment modality varies from person to person. Increased age should not mean increased anxiety. By addressing both the physical and emotional components of anxiety, we can alleviate suffering and restore quality of life. In this chapter we'll look at just what causes anxiety and talk about natural ways to combat it.

UNDERSTANDING ANXIETY

There are several theories on the causes of anxiety disorders. In fact, many experts believe that there are both physical and environmental components that combine to trigger anxiety disorders. Heredity, brain chemistry, personality, and life experiences may all be interrelated in causing anxiety. Particularly among older adults, anxiety disorders are closely associated with depression.

Some experts believe that a biochemical imbalance in our brains may lead to anxiety disorders. This certainly makes sense when you consider the strong relationship between anxiety and stress and anxiety and depression. But what these experts have yet to determine is the root cause of this imbalance. Does the chemical imbalance in the neurotransmitters of our brain cause the anxiety disorder? Or is the disorder present first, with the subsequent stress reaction of our bodies causing the brain chemical imbalance?

Individuals who suffer from anxiety disorders may have a brain chemistry imbalance resulting from a depletion of serotonin, as well as an excess of dopamine and adrenaline compounds.

Serotonin is an important chemical in the brain that regulates mental well-being and other brain functions, such as learning and sleep. Individuals with low serotonin levels are also likely to suffer from depression. When the brain creates serotonin, tension and anxiety are eased.

Dopamine is an intermediate in the synthesis of epinephrine, a compound that prepares the body to meet emergencies such as cold, fatigue, or shock. When the brain is creating dopamine, we may feel alert and think and act more quickly. Unregulated production of dopamine may produce symptoms of anxiety.

Adrenaline systems regulate important body functions like blood pressure and wakefulness. An excess of adrenaline production and release can take a toll on the nervous system. Extended states of "hyperarousal" and the accompanying release of stress hormones, such as cortisol, can wreak havoc on an individual's physical and emotional health.

While some doctors believe this imbalance in brain chemistry can be corrected through prescribing medications that regulate the transmission of these compounds in the brain, it is clear to me that the treatment of an anxiety disorder is more complex than simply prescribing medications.

Let's begin by looking at the types of anxiety and how you can tell if you are suffering from one of them.

Types of Anxiety

There are several types of anxiety disorders, each with its particular manifestation of symptoms. A single situation or event does not cause an anxiety disorder to appear. A combination of physical and environmental triggers can provoke any of the following anxiety disorders.

Generalized Anxiety Disorder

This is the most common anxiety disorder in older adults. Generalized anxiety disorder (GAD) is characterized by uncontrollable worry about one or more issues for a six-month period or longer. Chronic tension or excessive worries about health, money, family, or anticipated disasters are hallmarks of GAD. Women are more susceptible to GAD than men, and it is often linked to depression in the elderly. Physical symptoms may include trembling or twitching, muscle tension, headaches, irritability, sweating, nausea, hot flashes, light-headedness, and difficulty breathing.

Panic Disorder

Marked by intense fear and dread, this anxiety disorder is often accompanied by specific physical symptoms, such as chest pains, dizziness, nausea, flushes or chills, racing heartbeat, or tingling or numbness in the hands. People who suffer from panic disorder feel emotionally and physically less healthy than average and may suffer from alcohol or drug abuse.[3] If left un-treated, panic disorder can cause a person to avoid certain situations or events that make them feel anxious, leading to the development of phobic behavior. Panic attacks are more prevalent in late adolescence and adult-hood and usually recede with age.[4]

Phobias

Phobias are fears that have become extreme and irrational. People with pho-bias experience an overwhelming desire to avoid the source of these fears. This dread interferes with their ability to interact normally in family, work, or social situations. Physical symptoms of phobias are similar to those asso-ciated with severe stress: rapid heartbeat, shortness of breath, trembling, and an overwhelming flight response.

Obsessive Compulsive Disorder (OCD)

People who suffer from OCD have an uncontrollable urge to repeat simple actions, check things repeatedly, or have ceaseless unwanted thoughts. These obsessive thoughts intrude persistently throughout the course of a normal day, causing great anxiety and stress. Compulsions are acts that are performed over and over again in an attempt to alleviate feelings of discom-fort or anxiety. OCD is common in the elderly, and women are more likely than men to experience this anxiety disorder.

Post-traumatic Stress Disorder (PTSD)

This anxiety disorder is triggered by traumatic events that fall outside the range of what might be considered normal human experience. Survivors of war, sexual abuse, violent accidents, or near-death experiences may con-tinue to experience the resulting stress of these traumas throughout their lifetimes. Someone who suffers from PTSD may reexperience feelings of intense fear, helplessness, or horror associated with the event. They may suffer from nightmares or flashbacks. They may feel emotionally "numb," and withdraw socially. Problems with concentration, insomnia, and mood swings may also be persistent.

Diagnosing Anxiety Disorders

Late-life anxiety disorders can be difficult to diagnose for a number of rea-sons. Traditionally, medical professionals considered anxiety disorders to be less prevalent in the elderly than in younger adults. In fact, until recently, anxiety disorders were thought to decline with age. Research now shows that anxiety disorders in the elderly are indeed real and treatable. Data on panic disorders, OCD, phobias, and GAD indicate that anxiety disorders are clinically significant in the aging population.[5] Like depression, anxiety disorders impact women at a disproportionate rate: nearly twice that of their male counterparts.[6]

Diagnosing anxiety disorders in older adults is complicated, however, by several factors. As we age, we may experience certain medical conditions that may increase our worry about physical problems, and thus increase our anxiety.

Medical problems can mimic the symptoms of anxiety, or even trigger it. An irregular heartbeat can cause palpitations and shortness of breath. A clot in the lung (pulmonary embolism) may cause sudden, unexplained feelings of anxiety. Epilepsy and brain disorders may have anxiety as a symptom. Anemia, diabetes, thyroid disease, and adrenal problems—all may cause symptoms of anxiety. Even when caused by medical problems, anxiety may not always be relieved by the treatment of the underlying disease.

Depression and anxiety disorders are closely linked, particularly in the elderly. Commonly prescribed medications—used by many doctors as a first course of action to treat complaints they associate with aging—may produce increased anxiety as a side effect. Prescription and some over-the-counter drugs can also cause anxiety symptoms. Cold medicines, diet pills, antispasmodic medications, stimulants, digitalis, thyroid supplements, and, ironically, antidepressants may all cause anxiety. Withdrawing from certain medications, including certain blood pressure medicines, can also trigger anxiety.

Individuals suffering from the early symptoms of dementia, such as memory loss and other cognitive impairments, may suffer from a generalized anxiety, which can blossom into panic attacks. In this case, the panic attacks and anxiety may mask the true diagnosis of dementia.

Thus, to diagnose and impact anxiety in older adults, we must consider the complex relationships between anxiety and other disorders, and take a comprehensive approach that addresses the special physical, emotional, and social needs of this particular population.

Symptoms of Anxiety Disorder

In generalized anxiety disorder (one of the most common disorders in the elderly), the pervasive feeling of anxiety is associated with at least three of the following symptoms:

- restlessness or edginess
- fatigue
- lack of concentration
- irritability
- muscle tension
- disturbed sleep cycles

Individuals who suffer from anxiety disorders of varying types also report a combination of the following symptoms:

- unrealistic worries
- excessive fear
- exaggerated reactions to startling events
- "flashbacks" to past trauma
- ritualistic behaviors as a way to deal with anxieties
- shakiness or trembling
- muscle aches
- sweating
- cold or clammy hands
- dizziness
- tension
- dry mouth
- racing or pounding heartbeat
- upset stomach
- increased pulse or respirations

Acute anxiety disorders, such as panic attacks, may also manifest physical symptoms, including:

- hot or cold flashes
- choking or smothering sensations
- chest discomfort
- faintness

- tingling
- unsteadiness
- nausea

Identifying Anxiety Disorders[7]

Whether we are suffering from stress or anxiety, or caring for someone who may be suffering from an anxiety disorder, it is helpful to assess both the level of worry and the impact such worries are having on daily life. The questions below have been adapted from the Anxiety Disorders Association of America's Web site and may help you to separate feelings of anxiety from physical symptoms and determine whether you should seek help in treating a disorder that can become incapacitating, no matter what your age.

Circle the answer that best represents how you felt over the last week:

1. Have you been constantly concerned or worried over a number of things?   yes   no
2. Is there anything in your life that is causing you ongoing concern?   yes   no
3. Do you have a hard time putting worries out of your mind?   yes   no
4. Do your worries keep you from thinking clearly about other things?   yes   no
5. Do you avoid previously routine activities?   yes   no
6. Do you avoid social situations you used to enjoy?   yes   no
7. Do your worries seem out of proportion to reality?   yes   no
8. Have you experienced frequent weepiness, apathy, or unexplained weight loss or gain? (These symptoms can indicate depression, which is often accompanied by anxiety.)   yes   no
9. Were you exerting yourself physically when you noticed the chest pain?   yes   no
10. Were you exerting yourself physically when your heart started to race?   yes   no
11. Have you changed, or begun taking new, medication?   yes   no
12. Have you increased or changed your medication without supervision?   yes   no

Scoring Your Test

Give yourself 1 point for every "yes" answer to questions 1, 2, 3, 4, 5, 6, 7, and 8.

Give yourself 1 point for every "no" answer to questions 9, 10, 11, and 12.

If your score is higher than 4, you may want to talk to your health care provider about whether you are suffering from anxiety.

COMBATING ANXIETY NATURALLY

Success in treating anxiety in the older person depends on a partnership that includes the patient, their support network, and their primary care provider. Everyone must recognize and agree on the nature of the problem and make a commitment to stick to a treatment plan that addresses not just the immediate symptoms, but necessary lifestyle changes that will help the individual return to normal functioning.

Many doctors, once they have concluded that their patient suffers from an anxiety disorder, will probably prescribe a course of therapy that includes both counseling and drug therapy. Both of these approaches may offer relief from crippling anxiety disorders, but there are other treatment options that may offer the same results. For instance, in a Swedish study, a simple exercise program was nearly as effective in reducing panic attacks as any antidepressant.[8] If you are taking prescribed medications, even in combination with psychotherapy, you may find that your anxiety is not alleviated. According to Dr. Jeremy Coplan, a researcher at Columbia University Medical College, "Drugs don't work in a quarter to a third of cases." He further notes that this is ". . . exactly the same criticism directed at talk therapy."[9]

But when therapy and medications don't work to regulate the stress that can trigger more severe conditions, what can we do to protect our mental health? In the Mind Power protocol for impacting anxiety that follows, I recommend natural techniques for reducing stress and impacting anxiety. Changes in lifestyle, diet, attention to our emotional status, vitamin and mineral supplementation, and simple alternative treatments can prevent everyday stress from turning into crippling anxiety and control the symptoms of anxiety disorders.

Lifestyle

Stressful life events can trigger an anxiety reaction. Left unchecked, free-floating generalized anxiety can bloom into a severe and function-impairing disorder. By consciously making lifestyle choices that promote physical, mental, and emotional good health, we create a mind/body balance that allows us to access vital tools for preventing and reversing anxiety.

Exercise

Studies have shown that moderate exercise can release endorphins and natural cortisol, which act to elevate mood and reduce stress. Bodily pain and discomfort can increase anxiety in older adults, and gentle exercises such as stretching, yoga, or even walking can reduce discomfort while releasing stress. Exercise is also beneficial in normalizing sleep patterns and enhancing self-confidence. Choose a pleasurable activity and stick with it. It will not take long before you experience a positive effect.

Meditation

Meditation acts to calm the mind and relieve stress. Twenty minutes, twice a day, of mindful meditation is recommended to prevent and reduce anxiety. Engaging in breathing exercises and being generally aware of your breathing patterns throughout the day can be beneficial in eliminating anxiety. Focusing on the positive aspects of life and nurturing an optimistic outlook will reduce the effects of stress on the body and aid in coping with anxiety.

Cognitive Behavioral Therapy

For individuals suffering from anxiety disorders, cognitive behavioral therapy can help teach them to both change behavior resulting from anxiety and revamp their thought processes to prevent symptoms from worsening or developing. This type of therapy is short-term, lasting perhaps eight to twelve weeks. Goals of cognitive behavioral therapy include learning to identify behavior patterns, learning breathing and other relaxation techniques to prevent some of the symptoms of anxiety from gaining hold, and gradually becoming less sensitive to situations and thoughts that provoke stress and anxiety. It is important that a participant in this type of therapy be motivated to understand their behavior and work to change it.

Nutrition

What can be difficult in promoting proper nutrition as we age is the fact that our bodies may become less efficient in absorbing and utilizing key nutrients. Furthermore, someone suffering from anxiety may have little or no appetite or interest in food. Therefore, it is important that every bit of food you eat has the maximum positive impact on your mental health.

Foods and Anxiety

Studies indicate that a poor diet may be a significant factor in producing anxiety. To prevent and impact anxiety disorders, I recommend some very specific dietary guidelines.

One of the most important steps is the elimination of caffeine from your diet. Caffeine and caffeinelike substances found in coffee, tea, and many soft drinks can induce symptoms of anxiety, such as nervousness, fear, heart palpitations, nausea, restlessness, and tremors. Caffeine overstimulates the adrenal system and can deplete your body of important B-complex and C vitamins. The effect of caffeine has been specifically studied in patients with agoraphobia and panic disorders. An astounding 71 percent of the study subjects who consumed caffeine reported that the effects were extremely comparable to the symptoms they experienced during a panic attack.[10] A separate investigation showed that patients with anxiety experienced a degree of anxiety that directly correlated with their consumption of caffeine. Even more astonishing, this report suggested that the persons most at risk from suffering from anxiety effects have a heightened sensitivity to the effects of just one cup of coffee.[11]

Hypoglycemia (lowered blood glucose levels) is also directly correlated to anxiety and its related symptoms. Anxiety, sweating, tremors, and palpitations are some of the physiological warning signs that indicate our autonomic nervous system is sensing lowered blood glucose levels. Maintaining proper blood sugar levels by avoiding refined carbohydrates is essential to controlling anxiety.

Drawing upon the recommendations of Dr. Paul Epstein, a naturopathic physician practicing in Norwalk, Connecticut, and an advocate of a dietary approach to banishing hypoglycemic reactions, I have created the ABC approach to managing anxiety through diet:

- Avoid. Eliminate alcohol, caffeine, and nicotine from your lifestyle. Analyze your current diet and learn to recognize foods that cause distress. Eliminate these foods from your diet and replace them with foods that provide the body with optimal nutrients and support.

- **B**anish simple sugars from your diet. Sugar, fructose, glucose, corn syrup, corn sweeteners, fruit sugar, and brown sugar are the most obvious forms of simple sugars. Alcoholic beverages and many canned, packaged, or frozen foods are also high in simple sugars. If you do experience a hypoglycemic attack and must take a simple sugar in the form of fruit juice, for instance, be sure to couple the sugar with a source of protein (for example, beans, brown rice, nuts, or seeds) to slow down your system's absorption of the glucose and prevent rapid changes in blood sugar levels.
- Complex carbohydrates. Carbohydrates deliver the required energy more rapidly and efficiently than protein. Vegetable—as opposed to animal—proteins provide time-released energy.

Recipes

The recipes at the end of this book are intended to help you get started on a healthy eating plan that will provide optimum mental health benefits. Each dish focuses on foods rich in vitamins and nutrients beneficial to our brains. Eating right does not have to involve a huge effort. Prepare healthy dishes in larger quantities and store them for use throughout the week. In the list below are my recommendations for easy-to-prepare meals full of nutrients proven to help prevent anxiety.

Everglades Punch, page 258
Green Power Punch, page 260
Nuts and Seeds, page 262
Relax Your Mind, page 263
Sleep Insurer, page 263
Velvety Pecan Milk, page 265
Mixed Beans Vinaigrette, page 271
Mixed Sprout, Bean, and Nut Salad, page 271
Cream of Sweet Potato Soup, page 278
Nutty Banana Breakfast, page 281
Nutty Oatmeal, page 281
Indonesian Kale, page 286
Original Broccoli Stir-Fry, page 287
Pasta Fagioli, page 288

Sweet Kidney Bean Mash, page 290
Heavenly Roasted Nuts, page 296

Supplements

Even with a diet rich in recommended vitamins and minerals, your body may not efficiently absorb and process these necessary nutrients. As you grow older, your appetite may decrease, and you may find that you are unable to consistently take in the recommended amounts of food nutrients. It may be that getting these nutrients in supplement form is the most efficient way for you to enhance your healthy diet. However, supplements are not intended to replace healthy food choices.

Of course, before you begin any new health program, you should get a comprehensive, full-body evaluation performed by a qualified health care practitioner. A proper health and medical evaluation should evaluate your blood chemistry to assess your blood markers, your metabolic rate, and your blood pressure for indicators of cardiovascular, hormonal, or other imbalances or danger signs. If you are taking medications of any sort, for anxiety or any other condition, you need to inform your doctor of any supplements you are considering adding to your daily diet, as some may interact with prescription medications and cause adverse effects. You should speak to your doctor before adding any of these supplements to your daily regimen.

Vitamins and Minerals

Certain vitamins and minerals are especially important in fighting anxiety.

VITAMIN B_6 Vitamin B_6 is an important coenzyme in the synthesis of gamma-aminobutyric acid (GABA), dopamine, and serotonin—neurotransmitters that impact anxiety and depression. Research suggests that vitamin B_6 protects against neurological damage from hypoglycemia.[12] I recommend that your daily B-complex vitamin contain at least 75 mg of vitamin B_6.

VITAMIN B_3 (NIACIN) Nicotinamide (a type of the B vitamin niacin) has an effect on the brain similar to that of the class of drug known as benzodiazepines (tranquilizers and sleeping pills). Nicotinamide activates specific neurons in the brain, resulting in a calming effect, and can be beneficial in regulating anxiety disorders.[13] I recommend that your daily B-complex vitamin contain at least 200 mg of niacin.

VITAMIN B$_8$ (INOSITOL) Derived primarily from cereals and legumes, inositol has been proven effective in treating panic attack and OCD.[14] I recommend increasing your daily inositol supplement from 250 mg to 2,250 mg. Do not exceed 2,250 mg daily.

MAGNESIUM Magnesium is well known for its calming properties in persons with anxiety symptoms, but proper amounts of magnesium are generally lacking in the average American diet. Individuals who use oral contraceptives or diuretics, and who overuse laxatives, are at risk of magnesium deficiency. I recommend that women suffering from anxiety take a supplement of 320 mg daily; men should take a supplement of 420 mg daily.

Smart Drugs and Nutrients

A number of other naturally occurring nutrients may have beneficial impacts on anxiety.

ADAPTON (GARUM ARMORICUM) This naturally occurring substance is taken from a deep-sea fish. It is widely used in Europe and Japan to deal with stress, anxiety, and depression. It improves concentration, mood, and sleep. I recommend taking 4 capsules as directed for fifteen days; stop for one week, then continue with a maintenance dose of 2 capsules daily.

MELATONIN Melatonin is a hormone manufactured by the pineal gland in the brain. It is released into the bloodstream and is involved in synchronizing the body's hormone secretions and setting daily biorhythms. I recommend supplementing with 300 mcg to 1 mg taken nightly a half hour before bed.

THEANINE Theanine is an amino acid found in the leaves of green tea. It increases levels of neurotransmitter chemicals, including dopamine, which may explain its mood-regulating properties. In Japan, theanine is added to soft drinks and chewing gums for the purpose of inducing relaxation. I recommend taking 200 mg daily.

Mind Power Chart of Additional Supplements for Impacting Anxiety

The following chart summarizes the supplements I recommend adding to the protocol for overall brain health from Chapter 2. In some cases I will recommend increasing the dosage of a particular vitamin or supplement in order to specifically impact anxiety. In these cases, you should increase the daily dosage from Chapter 2 to the level recommended for this specific condition.

This protocol is designed for individuals who suffer from, or are specifically concerned about, anxiety. If you are concerned about additional brain conditions discussed in other chapters, consult with a health professional about how you can safely impact multiple conditions.

If you are taking medications—whether prescription or over-the-counter—or have any food restrictions, consult with your doctor before beginning any supplement program. Your health care provider should always be up-to-date on all vitamins, supplements, and herbal or homeopathic remedies you are taking. Supplement overdoses are rare, but possible, and certain combinations may affect individuals adversely.

Supplement	Dosage	Cautions
Adapton (*Garum Armoricum*)	4 capsules as directed daily for fifteen days; stop for one week, then continue with maintenance dose of 2 capsules daily.	
inositol (vitamin B$_8$)	Increase daily dosage from 250 mg to 2,250 mg. Do not exceed a daily supplement of 2,250 mg. Take in two divided doses.	
magnesium	320 mg (for women), 420 mg (for men)	May take six weeks or more for effects to be felt.
melatonin	300 mcg–1 mg at night a half hour before bed.	
theanine	200 mg	

Alternative Health Remedies

When suffering from a specific condition like anxiety, we can also try some natural treatment options that are considered "alternatives" to traditional medicine. While a healthful lifestyle and the proper nutritional and supplement plan are vital to winning the battle against anxiety, there are some other targeted remedies that might help, too.

Herbal Remedies

Some herbal extracts and homeopathic treatments have properties similar to conventional medications, but are gentler and may lack the drugs' side effects. Always inform your medical practitioner of any herbal remedies you may be taking.

- **Ashwaganda** has antistress properties. I recommend taking 450 mg twice daily.
- **Chamomile** is a gentle yet effective remedy for anxiety and the digestive disturbances that may accompany it. I recommend taking 650 mg daily, preferably with food. Chamomile may also be used as a tea, and is best taken in the hours before bed.
- **Ginseng** is an adaptogen that may help protect and strengthen the body against the damaging effects of chronic stress reactions. Do not take ginseng if you have uncontrolled blood pressure. If ginseng is safe for you to use, I recommend a dose of 200 mg per day.
- **Ginkgo biloba** increases blood circulation to the brain and protects nerve cells, and has shown promise in ameliorating mild depression and accompanying anxiety. Ginkgo can act as an anticoagulant, and individuals taking antithrombotic drugs like ASA, anti-inflammatories, and warfarin or Coumadin should consult with their doctors before taking ginkgo. Your daily supplement should be 300 mg daily in equally divided doses.
- **Indian snakeroot** (*Rauwolfia*) is a plant that grows wild in India and Africa and is used in impacting various conditions of the nervous system, including anxiety. Do not take *Rauwolfia* if you are suffering from depression. This herb is most effective when the whole herb is taken and used over an extended period of time. I recommend a dosage of 600 mg daily.
- **Skullcap** acts as a gentle sedative for the central nervous system. Consult with your doctor if you are taking any other medications,

including over-the-counter medications such as antihistamines. If skullcap is safe for you to use, I recommend taking 350 mg three times daily. Skullcap is often combined with other mildly sedative herbs, including valerian, passionflower, hops, and lemon balm. If you are taking such a preparation, follow the manufacturer's instructions.

- **St. John's wort** is very popular in Europe, where double-blind placebo-controlled studies support its efficacy in alleviating depression.[15] It has a calming and mildly sedative effect on the nervous system. I recommend taking 450 mg twice a day.

- **Valerian** is effective for people who experience anxiety-related insomnia. I recommend taking 400–450 mg daily. Do not take valerian for more than two consecutive weeks. Valerian is often combined with other mildly sedative herbs, including skullcap, passionflower, hops, and lemon balm. If you are taking such a preparation, follow the manufacturer's instructions.

Homeopathic Remedies

The following remedies may be used for both temporary and acute cases of anxiety. When dealing with a chronic condition, homeopathic remedies must be used in conjunction with other therapies, as prescribed by a qualified health professional. Consult with your health care provider before taking any homeopathic remedy, and follow their recommendation for the appropriate dosage. Always inform your medical practitioner of any homeopathic remedies you may be taking.

- *Arsenicum Album* is a remedy for exhaustion accompanied by anxiety.
- *Kali phosphoricum* is considered useful for anxiety and fear.

Acupuncture

By examining a patient's symptoms, appearance, and pulse, acupuncturists can diagnose and impact anxiety.

Acupuncture releases tension in the muscles. It causes a relaxation response in the body, resulting in lowered blood pressure and heart rate. Acupuncture increases the flow of blood, lymph, and nerve impulses to affected areas, and decreases stress while promoting feelings of energy and well-being. Acupuncture also is effective in relieving the physical symptoms associated with stress-related and anxiety disorders.

Therapeutic Touch

There is a variety of treatments that involve the transfer of energy from the practitioner to the patient that can help to relieve pain and anxiety. In one study, massage reduced anxiety and lowered saliva cortisol levels (a key measurement of stress).[16]

REIKI Pronounced "ray-kee," this method employs a powerful hands-on healing technique in which the universal life-force energy is channeled through the practitioner and transferred to the patient. Chronic stress and anxiety can deplete the energy in our bodies. Reiki is used to support the body's natural ability to heal itself. It releases spiritual and emotional blocks, and brings a feeling of harmony and vitality.

MASSAGE This popular technique can enhance general relaxation and provide an outlet for stress and tension. Massage therapy can reduce feelings of anxiety, promote better sleep patterns, and increase feelings of well-being.

SHIATSU This form of physical therapy combines traditional Chinese medical theory and various Japanese massage techniques. The therapist uses direct pressure with hands and fingers to redirect the flow of energy throughout the body. Shiatsu treatment is deeply relaxing and can be beneficial in both chronic and acute conditions.

Thought Field Therapy

According to Stephanie Marohn, Dr. Roger Callahan has pioneered a kind of energy therapy known as Thought Field Therapy (TFT).[17] TFT uses acupuncture points on the body to break up energy patterns that produce anxiety. By tapping on these acupuncture points, the energy is redirected and the pattern contributing to anxiety is broken. TFT is a self-practiced therapy that gives the individual immediate control in reducing anxiety in particular situations.

Aromatherapy

Essential oils can be used in baths or inhaled to provide rebalancing effects. Do not apply essential oils directly to the skin; they must be mixed with carrier oils. Experiment with some of the scents below to see what you find soothing.

- bergamot
- cypress
- frankincense
- jasmine
- lavender
- lemon balm
- lime
- neroli
- patchouli
- rose

SUMMARY

The Mind Power program in this chapter stresses the importance of nutrition and lifestyle modification, both in preventing and impacting anxiety disorders. Remember, anything that impacts this disorder can be used to prevent it from occurring. Anxiety has many causes, and the appropriate treatment will vary from person to person. What is important is to promote good physical health and a higher standard for one's spiritual and emotional life in order to combat the daily stresses that can contribute to more severe anxiety.

CHAPTER 5

MEMORY LOSS

P eople may joke about "senior moments"—those times when their memory suddenly fails and they are unable to come up with the name of their boss, or the time they are supposed to meet for dinner. The truth is, throughout our lives there are always times when our memory fails us. But because we have been taught that memory decline is a natural consequence of aging, and because we fear the onset of serious mental conditions—often related to advancing age, such as dementia or Alzheimer's disease—lapses in short-term memory as we age can result in ongoing stress, or worry.

Ironically, stress and worry are two factors that contribute to continued lapses in memory. The fact is, bouts of forgetfulness are usually unrelated to Alzheimer's disease, and there are simple ways to prevent and impact memory loss, and even maximize your memory as you age.

For decades, scientists believed that the health of the brain and our mental functions deteriorated as we advanced beyond our middle years. They told us that our alertness and decision-making abilities naturally decline as we move into the later phases of our lives. The accepted thinking was that the brain cells and connections began to die off as we age, and that this deterioration was inevitable and irreversible. We now know that this is not, and does not have to be, the case. There are significant data that shows there can be an ongoing regeneration and birth of brain cells throughout our life spans, well into our elder years.

This news should not come as a surprise. Goethe completed his great work *Faust* at age eighty-three. Michelangelo designed the dome of St. Peter's cathedral when he was nearly seventy. Winston Churchill, widely recognized as one of the greatest political leaders of the twentieth century, became prime minister of Great Britain at the age of sixty-five. The bottom line is this: the majority of people who live their lives engaged in vigorous and diverse mental activities remain neurologically robust, even at advanced ages. In this chapter I'll tell you how to strengthen your memory, protecting and maximizing its potential even as you grow older.

UNDERSTANDING MEMORY LOSS

Let's begin by taking a look at how our brains collect memories.

How Memories Are Acquired

The roots of memory have been studied and debated for centuries, yet many questions remain as to how the brain performs this basic function. What is known is that memories are constructed through a series of interactive steps that are triggered by exposure to new information.

Paul Scheele, the founder of Learning Strategies Corporation, a company involved in providing self-empowerment, educational, and health programs, points out that memory is not something that is retained in a particular part of your brain.[1] Unlike a computer, which can store information on a hard drive and return to access that specific information, your brain constructs memory from input from the entire neural network in your body. Memory is nonlocal. Each time you remember something, your brain is literally rebuilding an original construction. In other words, you can't remember something you don't already know.

The practice of construction and reconstruction is critical to memory. Scheele refers to this ongoing process as "mental hygiene."[2] Dr. Dharma Singh Khalsa, President and Medical Director of the Alzheimer's Prevention Foundation International in Tucson, Arizona, stresses the same thing when he talks about how important it is to "maintain the brain."[3]

Remembering something, whether it's the name of your mother-in-law's poodle, or how to dance the cha-cha, is a process that involves much of your brain. There are two primary types of memory, *declarative* and *procedural*.

The brain's medial temporal lobes, particularly the hippocampus, and the prefrontal cortex are responsible for maintaining *declarative* memory. Sometimes called *explicit* memories, these include facts, people, places, and things that we encounter frequently.

The capacity to learn skills or procedures, including new motor skills, is governed by our nondeclarative, or *implicit*, memory. This memory function is governed by brain structures outside the medial temporal lobes, including the amygdala, cerebellum, and motor cortex.

How Memories Are Lost

Scientists are unclear as to the specific reasons for age-related memory loss. It may be that our brain becomes less agile as it ages, or that imbalances in the system of neurotransmitters that communicate within the brain cause memory loss, or that other types of chemical imbalances in our bodies, such as changing hormone levels, impact our ability to remember things. What is known is that it is normal for anyone at any age to have lapses of memory, but that older individuals may face a higher incidence of memory loss.

Difficulty Learning

Studies suggest that the reason we have trouble remembering things as we age is that it becomes more difficult to learn new information in the first place. Memory studies have shown that about a third of otherwise healthy older adults have difficulty with declarative memory. However, a substantial number of eighty-year-olds perform as well as people in their twenties on difficult memory tests. Furthermore, all age groups retain newly learned information equally well, although it may take the older group longer to learn the information.[4]

Brain Circuitry

Brain researchers are not sure what, exactly, causes memory to be affected by aging, but for years they have speculated that changes may result from the subtly changing environment in the brain as it ages. Particular focus has been on the loss of brain cells and physical deterioration of the brain itself. But the role of an imbalance in the delicate systems of neurotransmitters that conduct all communication in the brain has been an area of recent study in relation to memory loss and brain function in aging.

A study in the September 2000 issue of the *Journal of Neuroscience* asserts that defective brain circuits could be more responsible for memory problems than the loss of brain cells.[5] Researchers at the Mount Sinai School of Medicine conducted a study that examined the synapses in the brains of rats and discovered that the ability of neurons to carry a signal was lessened in older rats whose learning ability was impaired. This reduced neuron activity was not correlated to age, but rather related to each rat's degree of learning impairment.

The Blood-Brain Barrier

It is important to understand the importance of the entire body's circulatory system in relation to the health of the brain. Blood carries nutrients to every part of the body, but the delicate tissues of the brain require a specialized security system. This tightly woven net of endothelial cells is called the blood-brain barrier (BBB), and acts as a filter, permitting only certain substances to travel from the blood to the brain. The BBB is responsible for providing neurons with glucose and other nutrients and also maintaining proper neurotransmitter balance.

The function of the blood-brain barrier is crucial, as it protects the brain from "foreign substances" in the blood that may be toxic to the brain; maintains a constant environment for the brain; and protects the brain from hormones and neurotransmitters in the rest of the brain.

The blood-brain barrier can be weakened in several ways, including high blood pressure; hyperosmolality (or high concentration of a particular substance in the blood); microwave exposure; radiation exposure; infection or exposure to infectious agents; as well as trauma, ischemia, inflammation, pressure, or injury to the brain.

Age-Related Alterations in the Blood-Brain Barrier

Studies have shown age-related alterations in the blood-brain barrier transport function, including a decrease in choline transport and a decrease in brain glucose influx.[6] Choline, one of the B vitamins, is critical in the manufacture of the neurotransmitter acetylcholine. Glucose is the primary fuel for the brain and supports many of the cognitive functions of the brain.

It is important, therefore, that the blood that is circulating throughout your body and brain is nutrient rich—full of the antioxidants, such as NADH or N-acetylcysteine, and the amino acids, like acetylcholine.

The Role of Hormones

Though memory loss affects both genders, it can be particularly devastating to women during and around menopause. In the book *Female and Forgetful: A Six-Step Program to Help Restore Your Memory and Sharpen Your Mind*, authors Elisa Lottor, Ph.D., ND, and Nancy Bruning[7] explore the uncharted waters that link memory loss to menopause. Estrogen has a powerful influence on the brain, playing an important role in functions like memory, language skills, moods, and attention. The authors describe case studies of women who, in the beginning of menopause, suddenly cannot remember simple things like their social security or phone numbers. The authors posit that the sharp decline in hormonal levels during menopause wreak havoc on memory. Fortunately, as the reported incidences of menopause-linked memory loss increase in scientific literature, so do the reported efficacies of treatment.

Diagnosing Memory Loss

It is difficult to know exactly when memory failure is a simple lapse on the part of your brain in processing known information, and when it is indicative of a more serious condition, such as dementia (Chapter 13) or Alzheimer's disease (Chapter 8). It is this uncertainty, perhaps, that makes these episodes of forgetfulness so stressful to the older population.

Let's start with the important distinction doctors make between normal, age-associated mental impairment and conditions such as dementia that signal a disease process. Not all memory difficulties or cognitive complaints indicate the presence of Alzheimer's disease, or other mental disorders. Many changes in memory or cognitive function in older adults are temporary and are linked to environmental factors, such as stress, or poor nutrition, rather than to physiological processes.

A doctor evaluating a patient who complains of memory loss will have to consider underlying factors, such as illness or medications, head injury or trauma, the possibility of stroke or heart disease, or drug or alcohol abuse. These factors can make it unclear whether their patient is suffering the "inevitable" memory decline associated with aging, or experiencing symptoms that indicate the onset of a serious condition like dementia or Alzheimer's disease.

Your doctor should also consider:

- essential fatty acid deficiencies
- chronic inflammation of the brain, which can damage cerebral blood vessels or neurons
- nutrient deficiencies

- hormone imbalances, especially decreased levels of DHEA, thyroid, and testosterone
- poor health habits, such as smoking, or drug or alcohol use, which can shortchange the amount of oxygen the brain receives
- atherosclerosis or heart disease, which can affect the amount of oxygen the brain receives
- brain neurotransmitter levels
- adverse side effects of prescription medications

Generally speaking, a memory problem is serious when it affects your daily functioning. If you sometimes forget names, you should not be worried—and there is much you can do to correct this tendency. In fact, researchers suggest that people who are aware of their memory loss probably do not have a serious problem.

If you have trouble remembering how to do things you have done many times before, or a place you visit often, or difficulty in understanding the order in which to do things (like following a recipe), your doctor should be notified.

COMBATING MEMORY LOSS NATURALLY

The good news is that the birth of new nerve cells in the brain is an ongoing process throughout our life spans. Rejuvenating your memory—or preventing decline in cognitive functions in the first place—requires a holistic approach to a healthy lifestyle that considers proper nutrition and beneficial supplementation, mental and physical exercise, and stress management.

We must reject the notion that memory decline is a natural consequence of aging. A person's memory should function at optimal levels well into old age. Simple memory deficits, if not addressed, can worsen over time. We must act *now* to keep our minds sharp.

Mental maintenance is a "use it or lose it" proposition. You must make a commitment to continually learn new information, to undertake new physical challenges, and to endeavor to remain open to new experiences. In the Mind Power program for preventing memory loss that follows, you will find the most important nutrients for your brain, the best ways to challenge your mental muscles, and the most effective ways to reduce the stress that can adversely affect your memory.

Lifestyle

As I said earlier in this chapter, we cannot underestimate the importance of the mind/body connection in maintaining mental sharpness. We need nourishment in all areas of our lives—physical, spiritual, and emotional—in order to prevent or reverse impairments of the mind. By concentrating on therapies and behaviors that improve circulation to the brain, rejuvenate brain cell metabolism, suppress free radical damage, and strengthen our mental muscles, we can boost neurological function and expect to maintain robust memory even as we age.

Exercise

The brain is nourished by blood, so it should come as no surprise that physical activity that promotes circulation is beneficial in preventing memory loss and mental fogginess. Changes in the body can adversely affect the brain, as one study involving male twins demonstrated. Tests showed that high blood pressure in men during midlife was a clear marker for increased brain aging, and led to an elevated chance of stroke later in life. The male twins with high blood pressure, when assessed twenty-five years later, had smaller brain volumes and increased strokes when compared to their twin brothers with normal blood pressure.[8]

The hippocampus section of the brain is vital for acquiring new memories. It is one of the select few areas in the adult mammalian brain that can grow new nerve cells. One study demonstrated that voluntary exercise increases neurogenesis in the hippocampus.[9] This was the first study indicating that neurogenesis can occur without learning enhancement.

Aerobic exercise, such as walking, gardening, swimming, tai chi, or dancing, has also been shown to sharpen memory skills.

Stress

Chronic stress—those day-to-day irritating occurrences that continue to build up in our bodies—causes the body to release cortisol into the bloodstream. Cortisol then travels through the circulatory system to the brain, where it begins wreaking havoc on the hippocampus.

As we age, our bodies find it more difficult to signal to the adrenal gland that it should stop producing cortisol. Prolonged exposure to stress then leads to the loss of brain cells in the memory center. Dr. Sonia Lupien, at

McGill University, has shown that the higher our cortisol levels are as we age, the higher the incidence of severe memory loss we suffer.[10]

Music

Exposure to certain types of music—especially classical music—produces transient increases in cognitive performance. The report examined a group of healthy elderly people and Alzheimer's disease patients to determine the effects of listening to an excerpt of Vivaldi's *Four Seasons*. The results of the study showed that listening to music enhanced the patients' ability to pay attention.[11]

Mental Exercise

The best way to keep your memory skills strong is to use them. Memorizing dates, lists, even telephone numbers can help keep your mind sharp as you age. The practice of construction and reconstruction of knowledge is critical to memory, so learning new skills stimulates your brain, too. A study in the January 2004 issue of *Nature* followed twenty-three healthy people (average age twenty-two) who learned how to juggle. After three months, MRI scans showed enlargement of the gray matter—the part that drives higher mental functions—in their brains. Learning a new skill had actually made their brains grow. When the study participants stopped juggling, their brains shrank again.[12]

Keep your brain entertained and engaged by practicing crossword or jigsaw puzzles, doing word search and brainteaser puzzles, or playing board games or card games. Learn a second language, take up a musical instrument, or take a college course online.

Providing your brain with a healthy body, good nutrients, and a stress-free environment is important. Challenging your memory and continuing the lifelong process of learning is critical to prevent short-term memory loss as you age.

Learning and storing new information may help prevent memory decline. Practice memory skills to enhance learning and improve your recall.

- **Relax:** tension and stress cause short-term memory failure.
- **Concentrate:** pay attention as you are receiving new information; you'll be surprised at how much more you retain.
- **Focus:** reduce distractions when you are involved in new undertakings that require concentration.

- **Slow down:** it doesn't matter how long it takes you to learn something; it's the acquisition of new information, not the speed with which you acquire it, that's important.
- **Follow a routine:** put important items, such as keys, in the same place each time.
- **Organize:** knowing where important information is can reduce stress; storing vital information in a visible place may be enough to trigger your memory without even having to look.
- **Write it down:** write down important things; keep lists.
- **Repeat:** repetition improves recall; use it, especially when learning names.
- **Visualize:** a strong link to a visual clue can improve memory; use landmarks to help you find places.

Nutrition

What can be difficult in promoting proper nutrition as we age is the fact that our bodies may become less efficient in absorbing and utilizing key nutrients. Furthermore, memory loss may cause you to miss meals or lose interest in eating. Therefore, it is important that every bit of food you eat has the maximum positive impact on your mental health.

Foods and Memory Loss

The nutrients present in the food you eat are the building blocks for neurotransmitters—the main network of communication in your brain. It's an easy correlation to make: if you don't nourish your brain with the proper foods, the health of the neurotransmitters will be compromised. When your mind suddenly goes blank, it may be that your lack of attention to diet has negatively impacted your brain's ability to do its job. It's a classic case of the domino effect, a perfect illustration of cause and effect.

A good maxim to remember is "What works for the heart, works for the head." When planning a brain-healthy diet, remember that, like your heart, your brain needs oxygen, it needs to be blood-rich in antioxidants and vital nutrients, it needs glucose for energy. Processed sugars, simple carbohydrates, fast foods, alcohol, and artery-clogging saturated fats are as bad for your mind as they are for your body.

Foods rich in omega-3 fatty acids—found in soy, fish, and other oils—as well as complex carbohydrates, high-quality proteins, and fruits rich in antioxidants, like blueberries, blackberries, and prunes, are the basic ingredients for a diet that promotes a healthy body and a healthy mind.

Recipes

The recipes at the end of this book are intended to help you get started on a healthy eating plan that will provide optimum mental health benefits. Each dish focuses on foods rich in vitamins and nutrients beneficial to our brains. Eating right does not have to involve a huge effort. It should be natural. Prepare healthy dishes in larger quantities and store them for use throughout the week. In the list below are my recommendations for easy-to-prepare meals full of nutrients proven to help prevent and restore memory loss.

Supplements

Even with a diet rich in recommended vitamins and minerals, your body may not efficiently absorb and process these necessary nutrients. As you grow older, your appetite may decrease, and you may find that you are unable to consistently take in the recommended amounts of food nutrients. It may be that getting these nutrients in supplement form is the most efficient way for you to enhance your healthy diet. However, supplements are not intended to replace healthy food choices.

Of course, before you begin any new health program, you should get a comprehensive, full-body evaluation performed by a qualified health care practitioner. A proper health and medical evaluation should evaluate your blood chemistry to assess your blood markers, your metabolic rate, and your blood pressure for indicators of cardiovascular, hormonal, or other imbalances or danger signs. If you are taking medications of any sort, for memory loss or any other condition, you need to inform your doctor of any supplements you are considering adding to your daily diet, as some may interact with prescription medications and cause adverse effects. You should speak to your doctor before adding any of these supplements to your daily regimen.

Vitamins and Minerals

Certain vitamins and minerals may provide protection against memory loss.

VITAMIN E In one study, researchers examined the possibility that vitamin E and other antioxidants could protect against neurodegenerative diseases.[13] The longitudinal study was conducted on 2,889 community residents, between the ages of sixty-five and one hundred two years.

Those monitored had their cognitive function measured by being told a long and detailed story and then being asked to recall items that were paired together. Those in the survey who had taken the highest amounts of vitamin E performed best on the cognitive tests. Based on the results of specific tests given the study's participants, the report concluded that vitamin E intake from foods or supplements is associated with less cognitive decline with age. I recommend increasing your daily vitamin E supplement from 400 IU to 800 IU. Do not exceed 800 IU daily.

VITAMIN C A powerful antioxidant, vitamin C plays a key role in maintaining healthy nerve cells in the brain. Vitamin C can reduce and reverse oxidative damage to tissues caused by free radicals. Vitamin C's immune-system-enhancing capabilities are also well known. It has the ability to regenerate oxidized levels of vitamin E in the body, thus enhancing the potency of that vitamin. In addition to your daily supplement of 500–1,000 mg, I recommend an additional 1,000 mg, taken up to twice daily.

FOLATE (VITAMIN B$_9$) A recent nationwide health and nutrition survey reported that grain products fortified with the B vitamin folate could help reduce memory loss in the over-sixty age group. A study linking the level of homocysteine (an amino acid found in the blood) with the level of B vitamin intake demonstrated that older adults with low vitamin B intake (in particular, folate) showed elevated blood homocysteine levels and suffered from a greater degree of memory loss than those with sufficient vitamin B intake. In fact, the participants in the study who had proper folate levels appeared to be immune to memory loss—even when their homocysteine levels were elevated.[14]

In another study, researchers at the Jean Mayer USDA Human Nutrition Research Center on Aging at Tufts University in Boston looked at the correlation between high homocysteine levels and memory loss. The subjects whose blood folate levels were highest seemed immune to memory loss, even though their homocysteine levels were elevated. The report suggested that consuming grain products fortified with folate may reduce memory loss in people over sixty.[15]

I recommend that your daily B-complex vitamin contain at least 800 mcg of folic acid.

LECITHIN AND CHOLINE Lecithin is manufactured in the body and found in many animal- and plant-based foods, such as eggs, liver, peanuts, soybeans, and wheat germ and brewer's yeast. It is often found as an additive in processed foods like ice cream and salad dressing.

Lecithin is a precursor to the neurotransmitter acetylcholine, and has a positive effect on cerebral and memory functions. Double-blind, placebo-controlled studies have shown that patients with mild cognitive disorders showed clear improvement when lecithin was given to them.[16]

A key component of lecithin—phosphatidylcholine—is broken down in the body and becomes choline, a building block of acetylcholine, a key neurotransmitter that plays an important role in memory. Levels of acetylcholine are known to decline with age, and studies have shown that supplementation with choline, which can also be found in liver, egg yolks, peanuts, cauliflower, soybeans, cabbage, and grape juice, can improve memory and learning. I recommend increasing your daily lecithin supplement from 1 gram to 2.5 grams for men and 2 grams for women. Take in two divided doses and do not exceed a daily supplement of 2.5 grams for men and 2 grams for women.

IRON Studies have shown that iron deficiency may be linked to problems with short-term memory. Iron is crucial in building brain neurotransmitter activity, and can be found in foods and supplements. Iron should be taken with vitamin C to improve absorption. Consult with your doctor about adding iron supplements to your daily regimen.

Smart Drugs and Nutrients

A number of other naturally occurring nutrients may have beneficial impacts on memory loss.

DMAE (DIMETHYLAMINOETHANOL) This nutrient, found in sardines, is a powerful stimulant that increases acetylcholine levels. Acetylcholine is an important neurotransmitter in the brain. It plays a role in memory, concentration, and focus. I recommend increasing your daily DMAE supplement from 150 mg to 650–1,650 mg. Do not exceed a daily supplement of 1,650 mg.

NAC (N-ACETYLCYSTEINE) This amino acid protects the brain from damaging free radicals by boosting quantities of glutathione, one of the body's most powerful antioxidants. I recommend a supplement of 500 mg taken three times daily.

NADH (NICOTINAMIDE ADENINE DINUCLEOTIDE) An enzyme that helps improve neurotransmitter function, NADH is present in all living cells and plays a critical role in energy production. It helps prevent cellular degeneration and may increase concentration and memory capacity. I recommend a supplement of 2.5 mg taken twice a day for two or three days of the week.

PS (PHOSPHATIDYLSERINE) PS helps the brain use fuel more efficiently. By boosting neuronal metabolism and stimulating production of acetylcholine, PS may be able to improve the condition of patients in cognitive decline. Studies have revealed that supplementing with phosphatidylserine slows down—and even reverses—declining memory and concentration, or age-related cognitive impairment in middle-aged and elderly subjects.[17]

As we grow older, aging slows the body's manufacturing of phosphatidylserine to levels that are detrimental to our functioning at our full mental capacity. For impact on memory loss, I recommend increasing your daily PS supplement from 300 mg to 400 mg. Do not exceed a daily supplement of 400 mg.

Mind Power Chart of Additional Supplements for Impacting Memory Loss

The following chart summarizes the supplements I recommend adding to the protocol for overall brain health from Chapter 2. In some cases I recommend increasing the dose of a vitamin or supplement from Chapter 2 to impact a specific condition.

This protocol is designed for individuals who suffer from, or are specifically concerned about, memory loss. If you are concerned about additional brain conditions discussed in other chapters, consult with a health professional about how you can safely impact multiple conditions.

If you are taking medications—whether prescription or over-the-counter—or have any food restrictions, consult with your doctor before beginning any supplement program. Your health care provider should always be up-to-date on all vitamins, supplements, and herbal or homeopathic remedies you are taking. Supplement overdoses are rare, but possible, and certain combinations may affect individuals adversely.

Supplement	Dosage	Cautions
lecithin	For men: increase daily dosage from 1 gram to 2.5 grams. Do not exceed a daily supplement of 2.5 grams. For women: increase daily dosage from 1 gram to 2 grams. Do not exceed a daily supplement of 2 grams.	Side effects may include nausea, bloating, vomiting, sweating, and diarrhea; extremely large doses can cause a heart-rhythm abnormality; do not use if you have bipolar disorder.
DMAE (dimethylaminoethanol)	Increase daily dosage from 150 mg to 650–1,650 mg. Do	May be overstimulating for some people. Headaches, muscle

continued . . .

Supplement	Dosage	Cautions
DMAE (dimethylaminoethanol) (*cont.*)	not exceed a daily supplement of 1,650 mg.	tension, and irritability may occur. Do not take if you have epilepsy, a history of convulsions, or bipolar disorder. If you have kidney or liver disease, consult your doctor before taking this supplement.
iron	Consult your doctor.	Have a blood test to determine true iron deficiency, as iron overload can cause health problems. Iron can interfere with a number of drugs, including thyroid hormone drugs, antibiotics, and drugs used to treat Parkinson's disease. Tannins found in coffee and tea can inhibit iron absorption.
NAC (N-acetylcysteine)	500 mg three times daily	Regular supplementation of NAC increases urinary output of copper. If supplementing with NAC for an extended period, add 2 mg of copper and 30 mg of zinc to your daily supplement regimen.
NADH (nicotinamide adenine dinucleotide, also called coenzyme Q1)	2.5 mg twice daily, two or three times per week	High doses (10 mg per day or more) may cause nervousness, anxiety, and insomnia.

continued . . .

Supplement	Dosage	Cautions
PS (phosphatidylserine)	Increase daily dose from 300 mg to 400 mg. Do not exceed a daily supplement of 400 mg.	

Alternative Health Remedies

When suffering from a specific condition like memory loss, we can also try some natural treatment options that are considered "alternatives" to traditional medicine. While a healthful lifestyle and the proper nutritional and supplement plan are vital to winning the battle against memory loss, there are some other targeted remedies that might help, too.

Some herbal extracts and homeopathic treatments have properties similar to conventional medications, but are gentler and may lack the drugs' side effects. Always inform your medical practitioner of any herbal or homeopathic remedies you may be taking.

Herbal Remedies

Some herbal extracts and homeopathic treatments have properties similar to conventional medications, but are gentler and may lack the drugs' side effects. Always inform your medical practitioner of any herbal remedies you may be taking.

- **St. John's wort** (*Hypericum*) is very popular in Europe, so much so that it is actually covered by German health insurance as a prescription drug. The recommended dose for combating memory impairment is 300 mg twice a day.
- **Butcher's broom** promotes healthy circulation to the brain, resulting in enhanced memory and clearer focus. I recommend two to four 425 mg capsules daily.
- **Chamomile** is widely recognized for its ability to reduce stress and anxiety, resulting in increased focus and concentration. I recommend two 325 mg capsules three times per day, preferably with food.

- **Eyebright** is excellent for impacting inflammation; its cooling and detoxifying properties may help with memory loss. Take two 430 mg capsules three times per day, preferably with food.
- **Garlic** cleans clogged arteries and increases blood flow to the brain. Add to your diet, or take prepared capsules as directed by the manufacturer.
- **Ginkgo biloba** enhances cerebral circulation, improves brain function and memory, and scavenges free radicals. Ginkgo can act as an anticoagulant, and individuals taking anticoagulant and antithrombotic drugs like ASA, anti-inflammatories, and warfarin or Coumadin should consult with their doctors before taking ginkgo. If ginkgo is safe for you to use, I recommend taking 40–60 mg ginkgo biloba extract three times a day.
- **Ginseng** boosts energy and concentration and may help protect and strengthen the body against the damaging effects of chronic stress. Ginseng can interact with many medications. Talk to your health care provider before supplementing with ginseng, and follow their instructions for use.
- **Gotu kola** improves memory and mental alertness. Elephants— animals known for their excellent memories—love gotu kola. Do not use gotu kola if you take medication for diabetes or to control cholesterol. If gotu kola is safe for you to take, I recommend 200 mg taken three times daily.
- **Huperzine A** sharpens the mind and wards off memory decline and improves cognitive and behavioral functions. I recommend 50 mcg per day with meals.
- **Vinpocetine** is a derivative of an extract taken from the periwinkle shrub. It enhances circulation to the brain and may improve mild, age-related cognitive impairment. I recommend taking 10 mg twice daily with meals.

Homeopathic Remedies

The following remedies may be of use for mild cases of short-term memory loss. When dealing with a chronic condition, homeopathic remedies must be utilized in conjunction with other therapies, as prescribed by a qualified health professional. Consult with your health care provider before taking any homeopathic remedy, and follow their recommendation for the appropriate dosage. Always inform your medical practitioner of any homeopathic remedies you may be taking.

- *Baryta carbonica* is for memory loss of recent events and general difficulty comprehending.
- *Lycopodium* is for loss of memory due to anxiety.
- *Argentum nitricum* can help a generally weak memory.
- *Anacardium* is for impaired memory that seems worse after a hot bath and better after eating.

Stress Reduction Techniques

Practicing stress-reducing techniques may aid in enhancing memory and focus.

RELAXATION RESPONSE One should begin each morning in a positive way, with some form of stress-reduction technique. Dr. Khalsa calls it "Wake Up to Wellness." Simply put, instead of starting your day with coffee, turning on the news, or reading the paper, you should start your day off in a positive manner. Find a quiet place so that you can practice some form of relaxation-meditation technique, which lowers cortisol levels, which improves memory.

MEDITATION Quiet contemplation allows your body to relax completely. Meditation can be done at any time, in nearly any place. Simply sit comfortably with your spine straight. Let your gaze drop downward, allowing your eyes to rest comfortably while remaining open, but unfocused. Allow your breathing to become rhythmic. If your attention drifts, or your eyes close, this is normal. Simply redirect your attention back to your relaxed downward gaze.

DEEP BREATHING After taking several normal breaths, begin to breathe more deeply with longer inhalations and exhalations. Breathe from your diaphragm—your chest will rise, your ribs will expand, and your belly will rise in sequence as you breathe. Breathe deeply and slowly, paying attention to each breath as you imagine tension draining from your body with each exhalation.

VISUALIZATION Use your imagination to recall successful or positive life events and link the feelings of those events to your present state.

PRAYER A way of getting in touch with our spiritual selves, prayer can take the form of silent meditation, affirmations, chanting, or traditional words. Repeat calmly, quietly, and in harmony with your breath.

Aromatherapy

Essential oils can be used in baths, or inhaled, or mixed with a carrier oil—like massage oil—and rubbed on the skin. Experiment with some of the scents below to see which are stimulating to you.

- rosemary
- peppermint
- frankincense
- rose
- clary sage
- geranium

SUMMARY

Diet, exercise, and stress reduction are all equally crucial in preventing declines in cognitive functions as we age. The Mind Power program recognizes that our brains are flesh-and-blood organs, depending on proper blood flow, nutrients, and mental gymnastics to keep them in peak condition. We are never too old to learn—and constructing an ongoing knowledge base is key in reconstructing important memories. Living life fully, both physically *and* mentally, is the key to staying mentally sharp as we age.

CHAPTER 6

MENTAL FATIGUE

If at times it feels as if the wind has gone out of your mental sails after you have worked too hard, in all likelihood it has. Imagine the activity of the billions of nerve cells in your brain as a steady breeze that propels your mental and physical boat. Sometimes, when the wind stops blowing, you can still move forward using the momentum you have already built up. In most instances, the wind will start up again before your boat stops.

When a neuron is stimulated, it emits an electrical message, and then it needs time to recover. While it is resting—a phase that lasts about ten seconds—other active neurons continue to transmit messages so that there is always a "steady breeze" of information flowing. Usually, the resting neurons are not missed because other neurons have picked up the slack. For a variety of reasons, however, sometimes too many nerve cells use too much energy too rapidly, enabling the brain to notice the gaps.

In this chapter I'll start by discussing types of mental fatigue and their causes. Then I'll tell you how you can implement healthful lifestyle and nutritional strategies to combat mental fatigue.

UNDERSTANDING MENTAL FATIGUE

Mental fatigue, also called mental burnout or brain fog, is characterized by symptoms ranging from forgetfulness to confusion, spaciness, lack of focus, and inability to think clearly. Unfortunately, often people suffer from these symptoms for such an extended period of time that they come to believe that having these symptoms is normal.

Mental fatigue can exist over extended periods of time, or merely be a passing phase. Both your physical *and* mental condition can contribute to a case of mental fatigue.

Types of Mental Fatigue

Your brain can become fatigued for a variety of reasons. When you have overworked your mental capacities, or when your body is physically stressed, your mental sharpness can decline.

Mental Causes

Just as muscles become exhausted after grueling exercise, the brain cells, too, can become tired when they are overworked.

HYPERFOCUS Unrelenting mental activity that is focused on one particular matter can exhaust neurons. Acute mental fatigue is fairly common among mathematicians and accountants after prolonged periods of working with dull facts or figures. Writers frequently encounter this conundrum, referring to it as writer's block.

INTENSE STRESS Essentially, whenever the mind goes into overdrive, mental fatigue looms on the horizon. A particular worry or stressful event can exhaust your brain and impact clear thinking.

MISUSE Investing mental energy in something that is against your nature can also trigger mental fatigue. For instance, if you are an honest person and you find yourself in a position that requires you to lie and, in general, become dishonest, then you are misusing your mind, and that can cause mental fatigue.

UNDERUSE Mental fatigue can set in when a task is repetitious and monotonous, requiring only rote memory to complete it. This form of mental fatigue is more closely related to physical fatigue.

Physical Causes

Imbalances in your body chemistry can influence your brain as much as your body. Several physical conditions can directly impact your brain's energy levels and ability to function optimally over time.

HYPOGLYCEMIA (LOW BLOOD SUGAR) Hypoglycemia arises when there is an unusually low level of glucose (sugar) in the blood. When the glucose level is dangerously low in the blood, it is precariously low in the brain as well. Hypoglycemia can lead to a lack of proper fuel reaching the brain.

CANDIDIASIS Mental fatigue symptoms can occur because of candidiasis (also known as a yeast infection or thrush), an infection caused by a parasitic yeastlike fungus called *Candida albicans* that is found in the intestines, mouth, esophagus, and throat. Normally this fungus is kept from overgrowth by naturally occurring bacteria (acidophilus) that are present in our bodies. When there is an overgrowth, there is a white discharge that can be itchy or painful. The overgrowth of the fungus can be controlled through diet changes, or medications can be taken to clear up the infection. Sometimes, mental fatigue may be the result of dying yeast. As yeast die, they have been known to release toxins that provoke temporary symptoms of mental fatigue.

CHRONIC FATIGUE Chronic fatigue syndrome (CFS) (also known as myalgic encephalomyelitis, chronic mononucleosis-like syndrome, chronic EBV syndrome, and post-viral syndrome) is a condition with complex, chronic, and debilitating disorders that has a multiplicity of symptoms. The cause of CFS is unknown, and there is no single diagnostic test. Some specialists link CFS to the Epstein-Barr virus (EBV), which is in the herpes family. Some authorities list possible causes of CFS as hypoglycemia, candida, and intestinal parasites.

FOOD ALLERGIES A food allergy occurs when the body responds improperly to a food or beverage that is not generally damaging to the body. Food allergies may affect your body and brain's energy production, leading to mental fatigue.

NUTRITIONAL DEFICIENCIES A diet lacking in necessary nutrients directly impacts the amount of energy available to the neurons. When your body is not receiving proper nutrition, your brain cannot function optimally.

Diagnosing Mental Fatigue

We have all experienced some form of fatigue. It is not hard to understand how running a race, playing basketball, or engaging in other aerobic activity can leave us physically exhausted. But identifying the causative factors involved in mental fatigue poses an altogether different problem.

Symptoms of Mental Fatigue

Mental fatigue, or mental burnout, is formally defined as physical, emotional, and mental exhaustion caused by long-term involvement in situations that are emotionally demanding. Mental fatigue is closely related to, and often interlinked with, emotional fatigue. They are both psychogenic—that is, states that are mental or emotional rather than physiological in origin.

Mental fatigue does not suddenly occur. It is a gradual process that takes place over a period of time. As the chronic pressures of everyday life mount, the body is placed under continual stress. We all know how damaging stress can be to our physical and emotional health. Scientific literature is replete with reports demonstrating how stress causes impotence, irregular menstrual cycles, heart disease, and even cancer.

Common symptoms of mental fatigue include:

- insomnia
- inappropriate drowsiness
- feelings of anxiousness
- feelings of stress
- loss of appetite
- inappropriate emotional reactions

Testing for Mental Fatigue

An indication as to whether you may be a candidate for mental fatigue is how you respond to the following questions.

1. Do you continue to do more, even when your resources are low or exhausted?   yes   no
2. Has your level of frustration risen so high that you do not see a way out?   yes   no
3. Has someone imposed—or have you imposed on yourself—unreasonable expectations that, because they are unattainable, have caused you to become sick and quick to anger at work or in your personal life?   yes   no

4. Do you feel stress shadowing you when you walk down the street, or do you see it staring back at you when you look in the mirror?   yes   no

Scoring Your Test

If you answered "yes" to any or all of these questions, you may be a candidate for mental fatigue or burnout.

COMBATING MENTAL FATIGUE NATURALLY

Once you have arrived at a diagnosis of mental fatigue, you cannot simply take an aspirin or a multivitamin or a nap and wake up relieved of your malady. Mental fatigue and burn-out are not something you can get rid of quickly, as you did not acquire them quickly. And because mental fatigue is so closely linked to disruptions in emotional and physical symptoms, you must take a holistic approach to restoring your brain's vitality.

In addition to examining the emotional and psychological stresses in your life, you must also look closely at your diet and nutritional habits. A hair mineral test can pinpoint nutritional deficiencies, metal poisonings, or other imbalances.

Mental fatigue affects millions of people. It causes accidents, crime, and problems in school and on the job, and interferes with relationships. That is the bad news. The good news is that there are corrective measures that can be taken to alleviate the problems associated with the condition.

In the following Mind Power protocol for impacting mental fatigue, I recommend natural, gentle treatments that will help rebalance the delicate chemical structure of your brain and revitalize your mental energies.

Lifestyle

Being aware of certain aspects of your lifestyle may help to prevent the symptoms of mental fatigue. Keeping your body and spirit refreshed will help your brain to function optimally and prevent mental fatigue.

Environment

Psychology professor Stephen Kaplan of the University of Michigan has extensively researched mental fatigue. He asserts that the most powerful cure for mental fatigue is the natural environment. One does not have to go to the suburbs to gain the benefits of nature. According to Kaplan, simply looking out the window and seeing a natural setting with trees and grass can reap rewards.[1]

A consistent body of research has documented the restorative value of nature in a wide range of illnesses, from recovering from cancer to keeping prisoners healthy, to helping AIDS caregivers with burnout. Researchers examining the biophilia hypothesis[2] (biophilia literally means "the love of living things") believe that humankind's relationship with nature covers a period of about 1 million years. If these researchers are correct, they are explaining why so many people thrive in a natural environment, but are ill at ease in large cities.

Exercise

Exercise improves your ability to think. Why? Even though the brain accounts for less than 5 percent of your entire body weight, it uses 30 percent of the oxygen in the body, and probably the same amount of glucose (which is the energy that runs your body). Quite simply, the more oxygen there is in your body, the more oxygen there is for your brain to use.

One recent study has shown that exercise may increase an individual's brain power. After placing twenty men and women between the ages of eighteen and twenty-four on a treadmill for thirty minutes of moderate to heavy running, the researchers measured the subjects' thinking capacity. When the subjects' heart rates returned to their normal resting rates, they were then connected to an electroencephalogram (EEG), an instrument that measures brain waves. They were then given two computer tests that were markedly different in their degree of difficulty. The results of these tests were measured against their previous tests, taken when they had not exercised in advance. The results were remarkable. They showed that when it came to decision making, exercise not only increased brain wave measurements, but, in fact, cerebral activity began thirty-five milliseconds (a millisecond is one-thousandth of a second) faster after the patients had exercised than when they had not exercised.[3]

Any kind of exercise you are able to do will benefit your brain. Walking, gardening, dancing, swimming, yoga, and tai chi are all excellent ways to promote both physical and mental health.

Nutrition

What can be difficult in promoting proper nutrition as we age is the fact that our bodies may become less efficient in absorbing and utilizing key nutrients. Therefore, it is important that every bit of food you eat has the maximum positive impact on your mental health.

Foods and Mental Fatigue

A good starting point for improving one's mental energy is improving one's diet. Organic fruits and vegetables should be incorporated into one's diet, while foods that cause allergies should be eliminated. While you are at it, get rid of junk food and too much sugar. Drink at least eight 8-ounce glasses of filtered or bottled water every day. Anyone with mental fatigue should not consume wheat and dairy. Foods that contain gluten—rye, oats, and barley—are also responsible for allergic reactions that may affect the brain. Certain vitamins and minerals can also help your body to fight the signs of mental fatigue.

To remain energized and functioning at optimal levels, the brain needs a full spectrum of nutrients, including vitamins, minerals, essential fatty acids, antioxidants, and amino acids. Deficiencies in any of these nutrients can upset the delicate chemical balance of the neurotransmitters and contribute to conditions such as metal fatigue.

Recipes

The recipes at the end of this book are intended to help you get started on a healthy eating plan that will provide optimum mental health benefits. Each dish focuses on foods rich in vitamins and nutrients beneficial to our brains. Eating right does not have to involve a huge effort. Prepare healthy dishes in larger quantities and store them for use throughout the week. In the list below are my recommendations for easy-to-prepare meals full of nutrients proven to help prevent mental fatigue.

Antioxidant Supreme, page 252
The Big Cleanse, page 253
Brain Power, page 254
Chilling Relaxer, page 255
Chlorophyll Boost, page 255
Delicious Detox, page 257

Supplements

Even with a diet rich in recommended vitamins and minerals, your body may not efficiently absorb and process these necessary nutrients. As you grow older, your appetite may decrease, and you may find that you are unable to consistently take in the recommended amounts of food nutrients. It may be that getting these nutrients in supplement form is the most efficient way for you to enhance your healthy diet. However, supplements are not intended to replace healthy food choices.

Of course, before you begin any new health program, you should get a comprehensive, full-body evaluation performed by a qualified health care practitioner. A proper health and medical evaluation should evaluate your blood chemistry to assess your blood markers, your metabolic rate, and your blood pressure for indicators of cardiovascular, hormonal, or other imbalances or danger signs. If you are taking medications of any sort, for mental fatigue or any other condition, you need to inform your doctor of any supplements you are considering adding to your daily diet, as some may interact with prescription medications and cause adverse effects. You should speak to your doctor before adding any of these supplements to your daily regimen.

Vitamins and Minerals

Certain vitamins and minerals are especially important in fighting mental fatigue.

CALCIUM Your body stores calcium in the bones and teeth, which is what keeps them strong. It helps muscles to relax, lowers blood pressure, reduces stress, and improves the quality of sleep. It helps nerve cells to communicate normally and promotes blood clotting. To perform these essential functions, the body simply takes as much calcium as it needs, leaching it from the bones. If there is too little calcium in your diet to replenish this supply, your bones will eventually become porous, weak, and prone to breaking. To safeguard your bones and prevent mental fatigue, I recommend a supplement of 500 mg taken twice daily with food.

MAGNESIUM Magnesium plays a variety of roles in the body. Not only is it critical for energy production and proper nerve function, it also promotes muscle relaxation and helps preserve the health of the nervous system. Magnesium deficiency may play a role in mental fatigue. Magnesium is also a building block for serotonin, an important mood-enhancing neurotransmitter that plays a role in reducing mental fatigue. I recommend a supplement of 320 mg daily for women and 420 mg daily for men.

POTASSIUM Potassium aids in converting blood sugar or glucose—the brain's (and body's) foremost fuel—into glycogen, a form of energy that can be stored in the muscles and liver and released as needed. Inadequate stores of glycogen lead to physical and mental fatigue. Potassium is depleted from our bodies in times of stress, thus upsetting the delicate balance of neurotransmitter communication in our brains. Potassium can interact with some drugs, so if you are taking prescription medication, consult with your doctor before taking potassium supplements. If potassium is safe for you to take, I recommend supplementing with 500 mg daily.

Smart Drugs and Nutrients

A number of other naturally occurring nutrients may have beneficial impacts on mental fatigue.

CREATINE Creatine was recently in the news because of its use by both professional and amateur athletes in bodybuilding, and evidence of its beneficial effects seems to increase daily. Scientists from the University of Tokyo reported that creatine supplementation (8 grams per day for five days) reduced mental fatigue when the test subjects repeatedly performed a simple mathematical calculation. Specifically, after taking the creatine supplement, those in the test group showed a task-prompted increase in the brain's utilization of oxygen.[4] Because creatine is naturally found abundantly in the brain and is an energy source for ATP synthesis, it makes sense that it should be effective in preventing mental fatigue. I recommend supplementing with 8 grams per day for five days. If mental fatigue persists, repeat the five-day dose as needed.

L-GLUTAMINE Glutamine is one of the most abundant nonessential amino acids in the bloodstream. It is produced in the muscles and is able to pass freely through the blood-brain barrier. Once in the brain, it is converted into glutamic acid and increases GABA, a neurotransmitter essential for proper mental function. There are two types of glutamine supplements: D-glutamine and L-glutamine. L-glutamine is the form that more closely mimics the glutamine in the body. For mental sharpness, I recommend supplementing with 500 mg, taken three times daily for not more than one month.

Mind Power Chart of Supplements for Impacting Mental Fatigue

The following chart summarizes the supplements I recommend adding to the protocol for overall brain health from Chapter 2. In some cases I will recommend increasing the dose of a particular vitamin or supplement to specifically impact mental fatigue. In these cases, you should increase the daily dosage from Chapter 2 to the level recommended for this specific condition.

This protocol is designed for individuals who suffer from, or are specifically concerned about, mental fatigue. If you are concerned about additional brain conditions discussed in other chapters, consult with a health professional about how you can safely impact multiple conditions.

If you are taking medications—whether prescription or over-the-counter—or have any food restrictions, consult with your doctor before beginning any supplement program. Your health care provider should always be up-to-date on all vitamins, supplements, and herbal or homeopathic remedies you are taking. Supplement overdoses are rare, but possible, and certain combinations may affect individuals adversely.

Supplement	Dosage	Cautions
calcium	500 mg twice a day	Take with food to increase absorption.
creatine	8 grams per day for five days. Repeat as needed.	
L-glutamine	500 mg three times daily	Take while symptoms persist, but not for more than one month.
magnesium	320 mg daily for women; 420 mg daily for men	May take six weeks or more for effects to be felt.
potassium	500 mg daily	Do not take potassium supplements if you are taking medication for high blood pressure or heart disease, or if you have a kidney disorder. Consuming foods rich in potassium is okay. Do not exceed a supplementary dose of 3.5 grams daily without consulting your doctor.

Alternative Health Remedies

When suffering from a specific condition like mental fatigue, we can also try some natural treatment options that are considered "alternatives" to traditional medicine. While a healthful lifestyle and the proper nutritional and supplement plan are vital to winning the battle against mental fatigue, there are some other targeted remedies that might help, too.

Herbal Remedies

Some herbal extracts and homeopathic treatments have properties similar to conventional medications, but are gentler and may lack the drugs' side effects. Always inform your medical practitioner of any herbal remedies you may be taking.

- **Rhodiola** *(Rhodiola rosea)* is a rose-scented shrub that has been a staple in Eastern European, Scandinavian, and Asian health practices for hundreds of years. *Rhodiola*—also called golden, or Arctic, root—is an adaptogen, which means it increases a person's resistance to chemical, biological, mental, and physical stressors. *Rhodiola* is a mild stimulant that boosts the brain's manufacturing of serotonin, an important neurotransmitter that helps you relax. Scientists have found that *Rhodiola* shows signs of effectiveness after just one dose, which is not the case with other adaptogens, such as Siberian ginseng (*Eleutherococcus senticosus*), which must be taken for weeks to be effective. A published report in *Phytomedicine* stated that in Armenia, a placebo-controlled, double-blind study of fifty-six night-shift physicians who used 170 mg of *Rhodiola* per day for two consecutive weeks stayed alert and had 50 percent less mental fatigue than those who took the placebo.[5] *Phytomedicine* also reported that in a Russian placebo-controlled, double-blind study, research was conducted on the physical and mental performance of forty medical students during a stressful exam period. The students that supplemented with 50 mg of *Rhodiola* two times per day for twenty consecutive days lessened their mental fatigue and need for sleep, and had exam marks that were 8 percent better than the other students in the control group.[6] For mental fatigue, I recommend a dosage of 500 mg taken twice daily while symptoms last.

- **Ginseng** is considered a rejuvenation herb. Research shows that ginseng is an antioxidant that slows the free radical damage of aging. It can promote better focus and boost energy levels. Ginseng can interact with many medications. Talk to your health care provider before supplementing with ginseng, and follow their instructions for use.

Homeopathic Remedies

The following remedies may be used for relief from the symptoms of mental fatigue. When dealing with a chronic condition, homeopathic remedies must be used in conjunction with other therapies, as prescribed by a qualified health professional. Consult with your health care provider before taking any homeopathic remedy, and follow their recommendation for the appropriate dosage. Always inform your medical practitioner of any homeopathic remedies you may be taking.

- **Calcarea phosphorica** relieves feelings of mental fatigue and forgetfulness.

- **Alumina** can help restore mental clarity.
- **Kali phosphoricum** is useful for nervous exhaustion and relieves mental fatigue.

Detoxification

Because the brain needs a substantial amount of blood, it is one of the first organs adversely impacted by the toxins residing in the blood. Metal and general body toxicity can contribute to mental fatigue. Toxic metals such as mercury can be found in our water, vaccines, dental fillings, food, soil, herbicides, and pesticides. Our bodies absorb these dangerous metals and our brain feels the effect.

When debris from the colon is not properly eliminated, the body absorbs these toxins, which causes the body to become poisoned. Brain fog, depression, and mental fatigue are some of the symptoms of body toxicity. The colon is not the only part of the body that is responsible for eliminating waste, however; the liver and kidneys also play a vital role. When these organs are malfunctioning, a host of toxic substances are allowed to remain in the blood.

Many people choose to detoxify their systems by following the cleansing plan below:

- Follow a two-week diet consisting of only raw organic foods.
- Drink ten 8-ounce glasses of water per day.
- Avoid dairy products.
- Use fiber, such as psyllium, each day.
- Use bentonite, a claylike substance that is used in a drink, which draws out toxins from the colon.
- Utilize colon therapy.

Breathing Exercises

Reduced oxygen to the brain is another common cause of mental fatigue. Shallow or interrupted breathing can be due to anxiety, stress, or illnesses such as asthma, bronchitis, or emphysema. Simple breathing techniques can help to relieve stress and tension. Long, deep breathing can increase oxygen flow to your brain and body. Alternate nostril breathing focuses your thoughts and concentration, improves circulation, and energizes the mind. Try both of the following breathing exercises to fight the onset of mental fatigue.

LONG, DEEP BREATHING Sit comfortably with shoulders and chest relaxed. Inhale, relaxing your abdomen as you push your belly muscles forward and fill your middle with air. Exhale, allowing your abdomen to shrink back in, tightening your belly muscles as you squeeze the air back out. Place one hand on your abdomen to feel your belly moving with your breath. Breathe in even lengths, breathing out for the same amount of time as you breathe in.

ALTERNATE NOSTRIL BREATHING Close your eyes. Press your right nostril closed with the thumb of your right hand. Draw in a deep breath through the left nostril. After taking a full breath, close the left nostril with the middle, ring, and little fingers of your right hand, taking the thumb away from the right nostril, and slowly let the air out. Expel your breath fully. Inhale through your right nostril. After a full inhalation, close your right nostril with your right thumb and release your left nostril and breathe out fully. This completes one round. Begin with three rounds of alternate breathing and gradually increase. Stop if you feel dizzy or faint.

Correcting Structural Imbalances

Believe it or not, the spinal column being misaligned, or any encroachment on the cervical, cranial, or other nerves, can result in mental fatigue. Something as simple as an improper sleeping position can cause a pinched nerve that affects the brain, causing mental fatigue. Chiropractic and osteopathic treatment and craniosacral therapy have proven effective in correcting structural imbalances.

Yoga and Meditation

Many have discovered the joy of yoga and meditation in helping clear the mind of thoughts that fatigue it. Brief periods of meditation throughout the day can help refocus the mind and reinvigorate mental energy. The practice of walking meditation is particularly useful for clearing mental fatigue, as it combines both meditation and simple exercise.

To practice walking meditation, focus your attention on each foot as it contacts the ground. When the mind wanders away from your feet or legs, or the feeling of your body walking, refocus your attention. To deepen your concentration, don't look around, but keep your gaze forward and soft.

Aromatherapy

Essential oils can be used in baths or inhaled to provide an energizing effect. Do not apply essential oils directly to the skin; they must be mixed with carrier oils. Experiment with various scents to see which are most effective at clearing away your mental fog.

- basil
- cardamom
- celery seed
- hyacinth
- lavender
- peppermint
- rosemary
- thyme

SUMMARY

Mental fatigue can be largely avoided, provided we pay careful attention to the amount of stress in our lives and strive to maintain a balance between work and relaxation. The importance of the mind/body balance is especially significant in overcoming the effects of mental fatigue. Proper diet and nutrition, as well as appropriate supplementation, can ensure that episodes of mental fatigue are brief and generally nondisruptive. By consciously seeking to keep our minds engaged but tranquil, we allow our brains to function optimally at any stage of our lives.

CHAPTER 7

PARKINSON'S DISEASE

After Alzheimer's disease, Parkinson's is the second most frequent adult neurodegenerative disease. Dr. James Parkinson, a British physician, was the first to officially describe the condition in *An Essay on the Shaking Palsy*, which was published in 1817. In all likelihood, however, the disease has existed for thousands of years.

A slowly progressive disorder affecting the central nervous system, Parkinson's is caused by the loss of the brain cells that produce the neurotransmitter dopamine. Without this vital brain chemical, the information transmitted on neural pathways in the midbrain becomes garbled and distorted, resulting in the breakdown of communication to the body's muscles.

What is amazing to me is that, for hundreds of years, doctors have taken notice of the initial signs of Parkinson's disease—a small tremor in the hands or a slight dragging of one foot—symptoms that are exacerbated when the individual is fatigued or under stress; they have learned that the absence of the neurotransmitter dopamine in the brain causes the physical symptoms of Parkinson's; but, tragically, after more than 150 years of desperately trying, traditional medicine has been unable to pinpoint an underlying cause or find a cure for this disease.

In this chapter I'll talk about the symptoms and progression of Parkinson's, as well as what modern medicine knows about this condition. I'll tell you what type of lifestyle and nutritional changes you can implement to help prevent the onset of Parkinson's. I'll also discuss supplements and alternative treatments that may help with symptoms of Parkinson's.

UNDERSTANDING PARKINSON'S

Parkinson's affects about one person in a hundred over the age of sixty—that's approximately 1 million Americans. Researchers estimate that this number will continue to rise, by fifty thousand or more each year, as the average age of the population increases. While certain symptoms of Parkinson's—lack of coordination, muscle tremors, and stiffness—are clearly physical, it must also be noted that over 40 percent of individuals with Parkinson's also experience serious mental decline.[1]

Although Parkinson's disease usually starts in later years—the average age of onset is sixty—younger individuals are not immune to the disease. When the disorder appears before the age of forty, it is called early-onset Parkinson's. In younger people who are afflicted, the onset usually occurs following an inflammation of the brain, as in encephalitis, or from poisoning by carbon monoxide, metals, or certain drugs.

You probably don't think much about the cause and effect of bodily movements as you go about your daily routine. It just happens. You want a drink of water, so you get up and walk over to the sink. To understand how the disruption of the delicate chemical balance in your brain results in the symptoms of Parkinson's disease, however, it is necessary to grasp some of the nuances involved in the functional relationship between your mind and your body.

In order for you to get up from your chair and walk over to the sink, your brain first has to go through a series of calculations that would be the envy of the most complex computer. These calculations involve accumulating all of the necessary information relative to the position of your body—the location of your hands, your feet, whether you are you sitting down, standing up, and so on. Once your brain has this information, it then assesses as much information as it can about where you are headed (the sink). The brain triggers all of the senses in gathering such information. The eyes relay information to the brain about whether it is day or night, whether it is raining or snowing, and how far it appears you must travel. Your skin—along with other parts of the body—assesses the temperature. Your feet ascertain whether the terrain is hilly or flat.

The brain gathers this data in the striatum, which is part of the basal ganglia of the brain. The basal ganglia are interconnected masses of gray matter located in the interior regions of the cerebral hemispheres and in the upper part of the brain stem. Basal ganglia affect normal movement and walking. Essentially this part of the brain acts as a command center for body motion. One type of basal ganglia, called substantia nigra, produces the neurotransmitter dopamine, which sends out the messages to the muscles that control balance and coordination.

Let's go back to the scenario in which you decided to get a drink of water. When you initially thought about getting that drink of water, your nervous system used the neurotransmitters to send messages to the muscles to enable you to do so. The role of neurotransmitters cannot be overemphasized. In essence, they are enablers—they enable thought to be transferred into motion.

As I hope the explanation above makes clear, dopamine is crucial in bodily movement. But there is another component to movement: *fluid* movement. Another neurotransmitter, acetylcholine, is invaluable in allowing the body to move fluidly. In order for the body to move smoothly, it is imperative to maintain the proper balance between dopamine and acetylcholine.

When a person is afflicted with Parkinson's disease, the number of nerve cells in the substantia nigra starts to decline. This leads directly to less dopamine being available in the brain. When this occurs, the delicate balance between dopamine and acetylcholine is thrown out of kilter. This interference causes a lack of coordination in bodily movement that manifests as tremors, muscle stiffness, and/or difficult movements.

Causes of Parkinson's Disease

While the symptoms of Parkinson's are generally clear, and the damage to crucial neurotransmitters eventually becomes apparent, there remain differing theories for the underlying cause, or causes, that may act as a trigger for the development of Parkinson's.

Dopamine Deficiency
Although there has been no conclusive underlying cause confirmed for Parkinson's disease, there is widespread belief that Parkinson's is caused— at least partially—by a deficiency of dopamine. In actuality, Parkinsonian symptoms are ascribed to a loss of cells in the substantia nigra region of the brain, which are responsible for producing this extremely important neurotransmitter. The parts of the brain damaged by this deficiency of dopamine are the parts that help regulate the nervous system and body.

A logical conclusion would seem to be that if one were to monitor the loss of dopamine, then the first sign of it diminishing would be an indicator of the possibility of Parkinson's. Unfortunately Parkinson's doesn't develop until 80 percent of the substantia nigra cells that manufacture dopamine are lost. Consequently, doctors remain unable to identify those in the early stages of the disease. Perhaps one day a test will be developed that detects the decline of the brain's dopamine levels earlier.

Free Radical Damage

Free radical damage[2] is also suspected of causing Parkinson's disease. (A free radical is an atom or group of atoms that has at least one unpaired electron, and thus is unstable and highly reactive. In animals, free radicals damage cells and are thought to hasten the development of cancer, cardiovascular disease, and age-related diseases.) Many believe that other causes—such as viruses or bacteria—are the principal threats to health. They are not. Free radicals are the principal threat to your good health, and controlling them may very well save your life.

Strokes

Interestingly enough, a person who suffers a series of small strokes can consequently develop Parkinson's. The symptoms in these patients are more likely to manifest as problems in walking than any of the other traditional signs of Parkinson's. In fact, the difficulties are more probable in the lower tremor and are more likely to have symptoms that are worse in the feet and the legs than in the arms. Traditional medicine treats this condition as if it were Parkinson's disease.

Chemical Toxicity

Pesticides and herbicides used on farms have been the subjects of studies to investigate a possible link between Parkinson's disease and long-term exposure to chemicals. Individuals who use pesticides in their homes are twice as likely to develop Parkinson's as those who are not exposed to pesticides.[3] Our food and water contain countless combinations of low-level toxic residues, and it is not fully known how these toxins impact the health of our bodies and brains.

A recent study in the *Journal of Neuroscience* demonstrated that the pesticide rotenone caused Parkinson's symptoms when given to rats.[4] The study indicated that the pesticide might cause the mitochondria to produce free radicals, and the destruction caused by the free radicals would subsequently lead to Parkinson's disease.

Metals Toxicity

High levels of aluminum, mercury, cadmium, lead, iron, and copper may also play a role in the development of Parkinson's disease.

- **Aluminum** is ingested from sources such as food additives, cooking utensils, antacids, buffered aspirin, nasal sprays, antiperspirants, automobile exhaust, soda cans, ceramics, and tobacco smoke. This metal is even found in some municipal water supplies.
- **Mercury, cadmium, and lead** are three heavy metals that can accumulate in the body with toxic effects. Mercury is a neurotoxin known to destroy nerve cells and cause tremors.
- **Iron** excess can intensify the symptoms of Parkinson's. Potential sources of iron include iron supplements, drinking water, iron plumbing pipes, and cookware.
- **Copper** levels can become high as a result of chronic inflammation, such as that caused by autoimmune or undetected allergy reactions. High copper levels, in combination with antioxidant deficiencies, can result in increased free radical damage to cells.

Bacteria Overgrowth

Certain bacteria produce toxic poisons called endotoxins. These toxins are released when cells die and cell walls become compromised. Bacterial endotoxins may flourish in the body as a result of the liver's inability to detoxify the system. When endotoxins reach the brain, they act as neurotoxins, producing acute psychotic symptoms in younger individuals and chronic nerve and brain degeneration in elderly individuals.

Diagnosing Parkinson's Disease

There is no known test that definitively identifies Parkinson's. It cannot be diagnosed through blood tests, or MRIs or X-rays, although these tests may be performed by your doctor to rule out other conditions. If you are concerned that you have symptoms of Parkinson's disease, you should immediately consult a trained neurologist, as there are many causes other than Parkinson's that are responsible for tremors.

While scientists have ascertained quite a bit about the symptoms of Parkinson's, relatively little has been learned about its cause and cure, and there remains little known about the risk factors for Parkinson's. Parkinson's disease affects both men and women equally. It knows no social, ethnic, economic, or geographic boundaries.[5]

Even today, doctors cannot recognize the beginning stages of Parkinson's, and there is a large degree of uncertainty in the diagnostic process that determines whether a patient, in fact, has Parkinson's.

For instance, side effects of prescription and nonprescriptive drugs (pain medications and selective serotonin reuptake inhibitors, or SSRIs—a class of antidepressant drugs effective in blocking the reabsorption of serotonin following the transmission of a nerve impulse across a synapse) can cause symptoms similar to those of Parkinson's disease, making a misdiagnosis possible.[6] These types of drugs may cause a condition called Parkinsonism, a nervous system disorder caused by damage to nerves in the brain. The symptoms closely mimic those of Parkinson's disease. If you find this hard to believe, consider that a study of autopsied bodies showed that 25 percent of patients who had been diagnosed with Parkinson's did not actually have the disease![7]

But there is no doubt as to what occurs in the brains of those who have the disease: the death and destruction of brain cells. An autopsy is sometimes the only definitive way to confirm the presence of Parkinson's. Lewy bodies (microscopic brain structures that may be observed in an autopsy) are an extremely strong indicator of Parkinson's disease.

Symptoms of Parkinson's Disease

Signs and symptoms of Parkinson's include:

- shaking (tremors)
- stiffness and rigid limbs (generally asymmetric)
- extremely slow movement (bradykinesia)
- impaired postural reflexes (extended arm tremor or trouble with handwriting)

When two of these symptoms are present, it is probable that the patient is suffering from Parkinson's. When three or more symptoms are evident, the patient is positively considered to have Parkinson's disease.[8]

Other, related symptoms may include:

- poor balance
- walking problems
- involuntary eye closure
- memory loss
- constipation
- sleep disturbances
- dementia
- speech, breathing, or swallowing problems
- stooped posture

Frequently, tremor (trembling or shaking) of a hand or a leg, particularly when the person is resting, is the first indication of Parkinson's disease. The tremor often begins on one side of the body (asymmetric), oftentimes in one hand. Eventually, a person's voluntary movements become increasingly difficult. For example, a once-simple task like walking becomes stiffer and slower. This is followed by speech difficulties (speaking in a hushed tone). Then the face becomes expressionless due to increased muscular rigidity. Since the person cannot control his or her facial muscles, there is often drooling. There may also be numbing of the hands and feet. Also, the person's handwriting becomes small—known as micrographia—and illegible. (If you have ever seen Muhammad Ali's handwriting, the first thing that strikes you is how small it is.) Although the person's thinking processes remain normal, they are stuck inside a debilitated body. For this reason, as symptoms worsen, a great depression may set in and lead to a shortened life span.

COMBATING PARKINSON'S DISEASE NATURALLY

As of now, we do not have a way to prevent the loss of nerve cells that produce dopamine or to restore those that have already been lost. Thus, effective treatment of Parkinson's would seem to rest on the ability to halt the damage to, and death of, the nerve cells that manufacture dopamine.

In fact, many individuals suffering from Parkinson's are prescribed the drug levodopa (L-dopa), which can be converted into dopamine in the brain. Levodopa is often used in combination with other drugs that appear to have protective effects on brain cells. Treatment with these drugs, however, does not completely alleviate the symptoms of Parkinson's, although the disease may progress more slowly. Long-term treatment with these drugs may result in neurotic or psychotic symptoms.[9]

Research is ongoing on the effects of other drugs and methods of treating Parkinson's, including a new generation of drugs that work to mimic levodopa and inhibit the enzymes that break down levodopa in the brain. Research is also progressing on surgical options, including a brain "pacemaker" that blocks brain signals that cause tremors. In late stages of the disease, some patients are treated with a surgical option called pallidotomy, in which a small section of the globus pallidus is destroyed. Some patients also undergo thalatomy, another surgical procedure that destroys a specific group of cells in the thalamus (the brain's communication center). Neurotrophic proteins and neuroprotective agents are also being studied, along with neural tissue transplants and genetic engineering.

Obviously, Parkinson's is a serious condition, and professional medical management and prescription drugs are crucial in staving off the progression of the disease and maintaining quality of life.

Recent advances in molecular science, however, are beginning to alter the diagnostic approach to Parkinson's—and the ways in which we approach treatment of the condition. Prior to these recent developments, the chief focus—and rightfully so—was on oxidative damage. Now, other causes—mitochondrial damage, excitotoxicity, and inflammatory cytokines—are being examined for the part they play in the death of brain cells.[10] At some point in the future, the chief cause of Parkinson's may be determined to have come from this group. But, as of now, any of these can lead directly to Parkinson's. Hence, the treatment modality should be multifaceted.

In the Mind Power protocol for impacting Parkinson's disease that follows, I discuss natural treatments that support the body and brain and are generally protective and supportive of good physical and mental health. Following this protocol may help protect you from the onset of Parkinson's disease, or help to reduce the severity of symptoms if you have been diagnosed with this condition.

Lifestyle

Although full-blown Parkinson's can be crippling or disabling, early symptoms of the disease may be so subtle and gradual that patients attribute them to other causes. Even if your doctor is fairly certain you are suffering from Parkinson's, there is much you can do in the early stages that may help to slow the progression of the disease. In any case, there are many elements of a healthy lifestyle that you can undertake at any time to help prevent the onset of a condition like Parkinson's.

Exercise

Exercises involving weight training have been linked to increasing testosterone levels that, in turn, elevate dopamine levels. Hence, exercising is crucial in fighting Parkinson's. Exercise also reduces stress, which has been found to aggravate the symptoms of Parkinson's. Specific exercise, such as that taught by the Alexander Technique, which focuses on ridding your body of harmful tensions through improving the mechanics of moving your body in day-to-day activities, may offer particular benefit to individuals suffering from Parkinson's.

Social/Emotional

When one first exhibits these symptoms, it is traumatic. Oftentimes, a trained professional's services are required. From a physical perspective, doctors generally treat the problems associated with motor functioning, for they are extremely alarming to someone who has never had sluggish movement of their limbs or rigidity. Though the patient is being treated for these physical symptoms, the doctor should also address the anticipated cognitive decline—for this greatly affects their quality of life.

Medications

Older adults commonly develop drug-induced Parkinson's disease after having been prescribed antipsychotic drugs, such as Haldol, Thorazine, Mellaril, and Stelazine. These antipsychotics are used to sedate nursing home patients with dementia and chronic anxiety, two nonpsychotic disorders. When these drugs are discontinued, most newly diagnosed Parkinson's patients return to normal.

Environment

Studies show that toxic pesticides routinely used in agriculture and lawn care are linked to Parkinson's disease. People tend to discount low levels of exposure, but in children, the elderly, and people already ill, even small amounts can be damaging, leading to any number of problems, including nervous disorders and cancers.

As mentioned above, heavy metals damage the central nervous system. Hence, it is advisable to avoid aluminum cookware, remove amalgam dental fillings, and stay away from cigarette smoking, for cigarette papers contain cadmium.

Nutrition

What can be difficult in promoting proper nutrition as we age is the fact that our bodies may become less efficient in absorbing and utilizing key nutrients. Therefore, it is important that every bit of food you eat has the maximum positive impact on your mental health.

Foods and Parkinson's Disease

A fresh, live-foods diet is vital to the healing process in Parkinson's. If you suffer from this condition, your diet should incorporate mostly alkaline foods, with green drinks, such as chlorella, spirulina, barley grass, or wheatgrass, once or twice a day.

Your diet should be rich in fruits and vegetables that provide a good supply of antioxidants. Antioxidants are critical for overcoming oxidative damage to the brain and for slowing down progression of the disease. Research has shown that a combination of antioxidants[11] can mimic chelating agents. (A chelating agent is a water-soluble molecule that can bond tightly with metal ions, keeping them from coming out of suspension and allowing them to be flushed from the system.) For maximum results, I suggest trying a combination of the C and E vitamins, polyphenols (found in green and black tea), bioflavonoids, proanthocyanidins (in grape seed extract and white pine bark) and curcumin.

Foods like egg yolks, red peppers, and onions that contain glutathione (a metabolite of the essential amino acid methionine) are thought to be beneficial. As are broccoli, cauliflower, brussels sprouts, and cabbage, which are rich in cyanohydroxybutene (a naturally occurring chemical that helps increase glutathione levels).

It is important to choose organic foods. The chemicals in nonorganic foods wreak havoc on our brains. Likewise, Parkinson's patients should consume only bottled or filtered water. Unheated extra-virgin olive oil and herbs for flavoring should be used.

Sugar and fat should be avoided, as research has shown diets high in sugar triple the risk of developing Parkinson's, while diets high in fats result in a fivefold increase in the odds of developing Parkinson's.[12]

You should also avoid wheat, dairy, and gluten products, margarine, fried foods, polyunsaturated oils, artificial sweeteners, processed food (such as deli meats), monosodium glutamate (MSG), alcohol (except red wine), and water containing chlorine or fluoride (remember, this not only applies to water you drink, but the water you bathe in; for best results, purchase a water filter, or be sure to keep your mouth closed while showering).

Do not use microwave ovens to cook your foods.

Individuals who are taking the prescription drug levodopa should limit protein intake to one meal per day—eaten late in the day—as protein hinders the absorption of levodopa.

Recipes

The recipes at the end of this book are intended to help you get started on a healthy eating plan that will provide optimum mental health benefits. Each dish focuses on foods rich in vitamins and nutrients beneficial to our brains. Eating right does not have to involve a huge effort. Prepare healthy dishes in larger quantities and store them for use throughout the week. In the list below are my recommendations for easy-to-prepare meals full of nutrients that may help prevent, or slow the progression of, Parkinson's disease.

Antioxidant Supreme, page 252
The Big Cleanse, page 253
Brain Juice, page 254
Chlorophyll Boost, page 255
Deep Sea Juicing, page 257
Fountain of Youth, page 259
Free Radical Delight, page 259
Green Power Punch, page 260
Head Cleaner, page 261
Pure Citrus Punch, page 262
Super Vegetable Cocktail, page 264
Four Bean Salad, page 266
Gary's Chef's Salad with Creamy Italian Dressing, page 267
Mixed Sprout, Bean, and Nut Salad, page 271
Succotash Salad, page 274

Supplements

Even with a diet rich in recommended vitamins and minerals, your body may not efficiently absorb and process these necessary nutrients. As you grow older, your appetite may decrease, and you may find that you are unable to consistently take in the recommended amounts of food nutrients. It may be that getting these nutrients in supplement form is the most efficient way for you to enhance your healthy diet. However, supplements are not intended to replace healthy food choices.

Of course, before you begin any new health program, you should get a comprehensive, full-body evaluation performed by a qualified health care practitioner. A proper health and medical evaluation should evaluate your blood chemistry to assess your blood markers, your metabolic rate, and your blood pressure for indicators of cardiovascular, hormonal, or other imbalances or danger signs. If you are taking medications of any sort, for Parkinson's disease or any other condition, you need to inform your doctor of any supplements you are considering adding to your daily diet, as some may interact with prescription medications and cause adverse effects. You should speak to your doctor before adding any of these supplements to your daily regimen.

Vitamins and Minerals

Certain vitamins may be beneficial in preventing and impacting the symptoms of Parkinson's disease.

VITAMIN B_6 Vitamin B_6 is essential in the synthesis of dopamine. When taken with zinc, B_6 can help stimulate the production of dopamine. While adding foods rich in B vitamins to your diet is fine at any time, it should be noted that when you use vitamin B supplements in combination with levodopa, the vitamin B may act to stimulate production of dopamine in other areas of the body, with less reaching the brain. Therefore, if you and your health care provider decide to try supplementing with vitamin B, you should take it either at the end of the day after the last dose of levodopa, or at intervals between doses of levodopa. I recommend increasing your daily vitamin B_6 supplement from 75 mg to 150 mg. Do not exceed a daily supplement of 150 mg.

VITAMIN C This potent antioxidant may help to slow the progression of Parkinson's symptoms. Ascorbic acid may also help to counteract severe side effects of levodopa. Vitamin C appears to be even more effective when paired with other antioxidants, such as vitamin E. I recommend increasing your daily vitamin C supplement from 500–1,000 mg to 3,000 mg, taken in three divided doses. Do not exceed a daily supplement of 3,000 mg.

VITAMIN E Vitamin E is a potent antioxidant. When taken in combination with vitamin C, it may help to slow the progression of the symptoms of Parkinson's disease. I recommend increasing your daily vitamin E supplement from 400 IU to 800 IU. Do not exceed a daily supplement of 800 IU.

ZINC A cofactor of vitamin B, zinc may help with control of symptoms, such as tremors and rigidity, and may improve walking skills and bladder control. I recommend a daily supplement of 30 mg.

Smart Drugs and Nutrients
A number of other naturally occurring nutrients have beneficial impacts on the symptoms of Parkinson's disease.

COENZYME Q10 (COQ10) As we age, our bodies' natural production of coenzyme Q10 (coQ10) diminishes. Our older bodies produce only 50 percent of the coQ10 they did when we were younger. This makes coQ10 one of the most important nutrients for people over thirty. Because the cells of our bodies need coQ10 to produce energy and to combat mitochondrial free radical activity, a coQ10 deficiency can result in a greater incidence of many degenerative diseases associated with aging.

Because coQ10 is a fat-soluble nutrient that goes into the mitochondria throughout the body, it should be taken with the fattiest meal of your day. When consumed in an oil-based capsule, the coQ10 can be absorbed through the lymphatic canals for better distribution throughout the entire body.

I recommend increasing your daily coQ10 supplement from 100–300 mg to 1,200 mg. Do not exceed a daily supplement of 1,200 mg.

DLPA (DL-PHENYLALANINE) DLPA contains two forms ("D" and "L") of the amino acid phenylalanine. The "L" form is naturally occurring and is believed to bolster mood-elevating chemicals in the brain. The "D" form is a synthetic form of a substance that has a pain-relieving effect. DLPA can stimulate the production of dopamine in the brain.

You should not combine DLPA with prescription antidepressants or stimulants unless specifically directed to do so by your doctor. If you have high blood pressure, or are prone to panic attacks, DLPA may aggravate your condition. DLPA should also not be used if you are taking levodopa for treatment of Parkinson's disease. Women who are pregnant, or individuals with melanoma, should not take DLPA. People with PKU (a rare, inherited metabolism disorder) should avoid DLPA as well.

If you are able to take DLPA, I recommend a daily supplement of 200–500 mg.

GLUTATHIONE A metabolite of the essential amino acid methionine, glutathione is an important part of the body's antioxidant defense system. Studies of the substantia nigra after death in Parkinson's disease sufferers have shown the depletion of glutathione.[13] To impact the symptoms of Parkinson's, I recommend a supplement of 200 mg taken twice daily.

MELATONIN Melatonin is a hormone manufactured by the pineal gland in the brain. It is released into the bloodstream and is involved in synchronizing the body's hormone secretions and setting daily biorhythms. It is one of the body's most potent antioxidants. In a study conducted at Thomas Jefferson University, researchers showed that melatonin was effective in blocking the oxidative damage in dopamine-producing cells, thereby reducing or blocking Parkinsonian effects.[14] To help ease the symptoms of Parkinson's disease, I recommend supplementing with 300 mcg–1 mg, taken a half hour before bed two or three nights per week.

NAC (N-ACETYLCYSTEINE) An important amino acid that enhances the production of glutathione, N-acetylcysteine can help protect the brain from free radicals and minimize age-related deterioration of the nervous system. I recommend supplementing daily with 1,500 mg taken in three doses of 500 mg.

NADH (NICOTINAMIDE ADENINE DINUCLEOTIDE) An enzyme that helps improve neurotransmitter function, NADH is present in all living cells and plays a critical role in energy production. It helps prevent cellular degeneration, and may increase concentration and memory capacity. I recommend a supplement of 2.5 mg taken twice daily.

PROANTHOCYANIDINS Proanthocyanidins (chemical relatives of bioflavonoids) serve to benefit the brain in a twofold manner: they are antioxidants and they protect collagen.

Research has shown that proanthocyanidins are fifty times more powerful antioxidants than vitamins C and E. Intricate tests prove that proanthocyanidins are great killers of the hydroxyl radical—the free radical that is responsible for the most damage—and lipid peroxides (rancid fats).[15] This is extremely important because the brain is particularly vulnerable to free radical damage.

Although proanthocyanidins can be found in the diet, the levels in food are generally insufficient to help fight the symptoms of Parkinson's disease. I recommend increasing your daily supplement from 80 mg to 380 mg, taken in three divided doses. Do not exceed a daily supplement of 380 mg.

Mind Power Chart of Additional Supplements for Impacting Parkinson's Disease

The following chart summarizes the supplements I recommend adding to the protocol for overall brain health from Chapter 2. In some cases I will recommend increasing the dose of a particular vitamin or supplement to specifically impact Parkinson's disease. In these cases, you should increase the daily dosage from Chapter 2 to the level recommended for this specific condition.

This protocol is designed for individuals who suffer from, or are specifically concerned about, Parkinson's disease. If you are concerned about additional brain conditions discussed in other chapters, consult with a health professional about how you can safely impact multiple conditions.

If you are taking medications—whether prescription or over-the-counter—or have any food restrictions, consult with your doctor before beginning any supplement program. Your health care provider should always be up-to-date on all vitamins, supplements, and herbal or homeopathic remedies you are taking. Supplement overdoses are rare, but possible, and certain combinations may affect individuals adversely.

Supplement	Dosage	Cautions
coenzyme Q10 (coQ10)	Increase daily dosage from 100–300 mg to 1,200 mg. Do not exceed a daily supplement of 1,200 mg. Take with fattiest meal of the day.	Dosage should be gradually increased, with 300 mg daily being added over a six-week period until the daily dose reaches 1,200 mg. Individuals supplementing with coQ10 at high doses should be monitored closely by their doctors.
DLPA (DL-phenylalanine)	200–500 mg daily	Contraindicated for use with levodopa and MAOs. Consult with your doctor before taking. Individuals with certain mental health problems should not take this supplement.
glutathione	200 mg two times daily	Glutathione levels may also be elevated through supplementation with cysteine, N-acetylcysteine, or L-cysteine.
melatonin	300 mcg–1 mg two to three nights per week a half hour before bed	Tolerance may develop with regular use. Long-term effects of nightly use are unknown.
N-acetylcysteine	1,500 mg in three divided doses	Regular supplementation of NAC increases urinary output of copper. If supplementing with NAC for an extended period, add

Supplement	Dosage	Cautions
N-acetylcysteine (*cont.*)		2 mg of copper and 30 mg of zinc to your daily supplement regimen.
NADH (nicotinamide adenine dinucleotide)	2.5 mg twice daily	High doses (10 mg per day or more) may cause nervousness, anxiety, and insomnia.
proanthocyanidins	Increase daily dosage from 80 mg to 380 mg, taken in three divided doses. Do not exceed a daily supplement of 380 mg.	
vitamin B$_6$	Increase daily dosage from 75 mg to 150 mg. Do not exceed a daily supplement of 150 mg. Take with zinc (30 mg).	Contraindicated for use with levodopa. Discuss supplementation with your health care provider.
vitamin C	Increase daily dosage from 500–1,000 mg to 3,000 mg, taken in three divided doses. Do not exceed a daily supplement of 3,000 mg.	
vitamin E	Increase daily dosage from 400 IU to 800 IU. Do not exceed a daily supplement of 800 IU.	If you have high blood pressure, limit your supplemental vitamin E to 400 IU daily. If you are taking blood thinners, consult with your doctor before taking vitamin E.
zinc	Up to 30 mg daily	Large doses (50 mg or more) can interfere with the body's absorption of essential minerals, impair blood cell function, and depress immune system.

Alternative Health Remedies

When suffering from a specific condition like Parkinson's disease, we can also try some natural treatment options that are considered "alternatives" to traditional medicine. While a healthful lifestyle and the proper nutritional and supplement plan are vital to winning the battle against the symptoms of Parkinson's, there are some other targeted remedies that might help, too.

Herbal Remedies

Some herbal extracts and homeopathic treatments have properties similar to conventional medications, but are gentler and may lack the drugs' side effects. Always inform your medical practitioner of any herbal remedies you may be taking.

- **Atmagupta** *(Mucuna pruriens)* is an Ayurvedic herb that contains the natural form of L-dopa. Ayurvedic herbs are commonly taken in combination to neutralize toxicity. Do not take this without consulting with your doctor.
- **Gotu kola** has been historically used in the treatment of Parkinson's disease. I recommend taking it as a tea once daily. Do not use gotu kola if you take medication for diabetes or to control cholesterol. If gotu kola is safe for you to take, I recommend 200 mg taken three times daily.
- **Ginkgo biloba** is an extract of the ginkgo plant used in Europe to help fight dementia and Alzheimer's disease. It is a circulatory stimulant and an antioxidant. Ginkgo can act as an anticoagulant, and individuals taking anticoagulant and antithrombotic drugs like ASA, anti-inflammatories, and warfarin or Coumadin should consult with their doctor before taking ginkgo. If ginkgo is safe for you to use, I recommend a supplement of 120 mg per day taken in three equal doses.
- **Hawthorn** acts as a circulatory stimulant and potent antioxidant. I recommend a supplement of 2–5 grams per day.
- **Lady's slipper** may help provide relief from tremors. I recommend 10–30 drops of tincture taken three or four times daily.
- **Milk thistle** can provide liver support and detoxification. I recommend a supplement of 30–60 drops of tincture per day.
- **Skullcap** acts to strengthen the brain. I recommend 10–30 drops of tincture per day.

Homeopathic Remedies

The following remedies may be used for relief from the symptoms of Parkinson's disease. When dealing with a chronic condition, homeopathic remedies must be used in conjunction with other therapies, as prescribed by a qualified health professional. Consult with your health care provider before taking any homeopathic remedy, and follow their recommendation for the appropriate dosage. Always inform your medical practitioner of any homeopathic remedies you may be taking.

- **Anthimonium tartaricum** may help with trembling head and immobile hands.
- **Gelsemium** may provide relief from trembling and drooping eyelids.
- **Agarius** is for limbs that are stiff but tremble and twitch; your back and spine may be especially sensitive.
- **Rhus toxicodendron** is good for mild tremors and stiffness that feels better after movement, worse with damp weather.

Detoxification

Chelation therapy eliminates metals from the brain, as well as other toxic agents that encourage free radicals' development. A hair analysis can determine whether high levels of metals need to be chelated out of the body. Studies indicate that to properly impact Parkinson's, effective treatments must reduce oxidative stress. Chelation therapy plays an important role in eliminating iron as well as other toxins from the brain. These toxins infuse the brain with free radicals. Some think that chelation can only occur through chelation therapy. Antioxidants can also play the role of chelators, however. The C and E vitamins, bioflavonoids, polyphenols (from black and green teas), grape seed extract (specifically, the proanthocyanidins), and tocotrienols from curcumin also serve as chelators. To find out more about chelation therapy and detoxification protocols, visit my Web site: www.garynull.com.

Aromatherapy

Essential oils can be used in baths or inhaled to provide rebalancing effects. Do not apply essential oils directly to the skin; they must be mixed with carrier oils. Though massaging with fragrant essential oils will not cure Parkinson's, it can provide temporary relief. Experiment with various scents to see which brings you relief.

- clary sage
- marjoram
- lavender

SUMMARY

Keep in mind that conventional medicine has defined Parkinson's as a disease that cannot be reversed. Alternative and complementary medicine has demonstrated otherwise. The Mind Power protocol for Parkinson's can help protect your brain and offer relief from the progression of the symptoms of this disease.

CHAPTER 8

ALZHEIMER'S DISEASE

When I speak to people about some of the serious conditions associated with aging, the same concern comes up over and over again: "Gary, my father [or mother, or grandparent] suffered from Alzheimer's. Is there anything I can do to keep from getting this disease as I grow older?"

Alzheimer's disease is one of the most dreaded of the numerous mental disorders associated with aging. Its slow, progressive assault on an individual's mental function robs sufferers of their memory—and often their dignity. Alzheimer's advances in stages, first causing disturbances in verbal, then visual, memory before destroying the brain's executive functions, causing loss of ability to reason, plan, or organize thoughts, loss of language, and inability to recognize objects.

The severe memory impairment—or dementia—that occurs with Alzheimer's disease significantly interferes with daily life. Simple tasks become difficult or impossible to perform, and day-to-day functioning becomes increasingly diminished. But Alzheimer's is not a normal part of the aging process. And even if there is a history of the disease in your family, it is not inevitable that you will suffer its effects as you age.

By providing an optimal environment for brain health, through a healthful lifestyle, attention to nutrition, and proper supplementation, you can preserve your mental abilities as you age. In this chapter I will talk about specific steps you can take to improve your environment and diet to protect your brain against the symptoms of cognitive decline associated with Alzheimer's. I will also talk about alternative, natural treatments that may have some benefits in the fight against this serious condition.

UNDERSTANDING ALZHEIMER'S DISEASE

According to the Alzheimer's Association,[1] Alzheimer's disease now affects approximately 4.5 million Americans. In a Gallup poll commissioned by the Alzheimer's Association, one in ten Americans said they had a family member with Alzheimer's disease and one in three knew someone with the disease. As the number of Americans with this condition continues to grow, it is projected that by 2050 the number of individuals with Alzheimer's could range from 11.3 million to 16 million.

Alzheimer's is one form of dementia—a term used to describe a group of symptoms that are caused by changes in brain function. Many different conditions can cause symptoms that mimic those of Alzheimer's disease but are not Alzheimer's. In fact, Alzheimer's has a specific, visible effect on the physical condition of the brain as neurons, specifically those in the hippocampus, progressively degenerate, lose function, and die.

The German physician Alois Alzheimer first discovered this physical change in the brain in 1906. He presented his findings on the brain condition of a woman who had died while suffering from a rare mental disease that caused loss of memory, confusion, and hallucination before her death at age fifty-five. He described these changes in the brain as atypical clumps and twisted bundles of neurofibers accompanied by cell death as evidenced by shrinkage in the brain.

Nearly a century later, the cause of this cell death remains the subject of intense scientific scrutiny, which has provided clues, but few conclusions. Many experts believe that the cell death is related to a sticky, waxy protein called amyloid plaque, but whether the plaque causes cell death or is a byproduct of it is unclear.

A second feature of Alzheimer's disease is neurofibrillary tangles consisting of tau protein (an essential protein in the infrastructure of neurons). When the tau protein disintegrates, it coils into filaments that gather in tangles. These plaques and tangles disrupt the communication in the brain, obstructing the electrical messages sent from neuron to neuron that allow us to think, remember, talk, and move.

As neurons begin to die, the amount of acetylcholine, a crucial chemical in the brain, decreases. Acetylcholine is necessary to carry the complex messages governing reactions and movement. Thus, as Alzheimer's progresses, physical impairment begins to occur along with cognitive losses.

Causes of Alzheimer's Disease

Doctors remain unable to state with certainty the cause of Alzheimer's disease. While there is no definitive cause of Alzheimer's disease, there are certain risk factors that may increase your chances of becoming a victim of this serious form of dementia. There are many health professionals who hypothesize that Alzheimer's is the result of a combination of factors. As you look at the various risk criteria outlined below, it is worth noting that many of them can be proactively addressed.

Chemical Risk Factors

Imbalances in your body's delicate network of neurotransmitters, nutrient deficiencies, and metabolic deficits have all been implicated in the development and progression of the symptoms of Alzheimer's disease.

- **Hyperhomocysteinemia,** or high homocysteine levels, is significantly correlated with low levels of the nutrients folic acid and vitamins B_6 and B_{12}.
- **Altered taurine metabolism**—the body's ability to metabolize taurine, a nonessential amino acid necessary for the proper development and maintenance of the central nervous system—may contribute to the memory loss that is characteristic of Alzheimer's when altered.
- **Low levels of DHEA,** an adrenal hormone that declines with age.
- **Low levels of acetylcholine, serotonin, GABA, dopamine, and norepinephrine,** which are all key neurotransmitters.
- **Estrogen imbalance.**

Environmental Risk Factors

External factors may play a role in the development and progression of symptoms of Alzheimer's disease. Such factors include: exposures to neurotoxins, such as mercury, lead, pesticides, and excess iron; alcohol abuse; free radical damage; and aluminum exposure.

Social Risk Factors

Factors such as lower levels of education, lack of social contact, poor word fluency, emotional stress and/or poor stress coping mechanisms, and the lack of willingness to learn new information and face mental challenges have all been implicated in the development and progression of the symptoms of Alzheimer's disease.

Physical Risk Factors

Possible physical risk factors include advanced age, a history of Parkinson's disease or Down's syndrome, head trauma, depression, reduced blood flow, stroke, olfactory deficits, gum disease or other markers for inflammation, or coronary disease.

Diagnosing Alzheimer's Disease

The presence of amyloid plaques and neurofibrillary tangles are the only definitive way to make a positive diagnosis of Alzheimer's disease. Progress is being made in using advanced imaging technologies and novel biomarkers to detect Alzheimer's disease and dementia before they reach the moderate stages. Unfortunately, even the powerful imaging tools used by doctors today cannot reliably scan for these markers. Only a brain biopsy or an autopsy can provide positive confirmation that Alzheimer's disease is the cause of an individual's dementia.

Because Alzheimer's is so common in the aging population, the medical profession has established some general protocols to arrive at a clinical diagnosis of Alzheimer's. By relying on a process of elimination, doctors rule out other possible causes of symptoms of cognitive failure.

Early detection of Alzheimer's disease is extremely difficult. Most clinical diagnoses are made in patients who have already developed a considerable amount of mental difficulties. Furthermore, the earliest signs of Alzheimer's disease can be extremely difficult to self-detect.

Stages of Alzheimer's Disease[2]

Experts have documented common patterns in the progression of symptoms of individuals with Alzheimer's disease and have created a system of "staging" the disease as it unfolds. The seven stages range from "no impairment" to "very severe decline." Stages 2 through 4 are considered early-stage; stages 5 and 6 are considered mid-stage, and stage 7 is considered late-stage Alzheimer's.

- **Stage 1.** No cognitive impairment.
- **Stage 2.** Very mild cognitive decline marked by memory lapses,

especially forgetting familiar words or names, or the location of every-day objects. Not generally apparent to friends, family, or coworkers.

- **Stage 3.** Mild cognitive decline that is noticeable to friends, family, or coworkers. Common difficulties may include problems remembering familiar names, decreased ability to remember new information, performance issues in work or social situations, inability to retain information, losing or misplacing valuable objects, and decline in ability to plan or organize.

- **Stage 4.** Moderate cognitive decline with clear-cut deficiencies, including: decreased knowledge of recent occasions or current events; impaired ability to perform challenging mental exercises (for example, counting backward from 100 by 7s); decreased ability to perform complex tasks, like bill paying, managing finances, or grocery shopping; reduced memory of personal history; and appearing subdued and withdrawn, especially in socially or mentally challenging situations.

- **Stage 5.** Moderately severe cognitive decline with major gaps in memory and deficits in cognitive function, including the inability to recall important details, such as address or phone number; confusion about days, dates, and the season; difficulty with less challenging mental exercises (for example, counting backward from 20 by 2s); and difficulty with performing abstract reasoning tasks, such as dressing appropriately for the season.

- **Stage 6.** Severe cognitive decline marked by worsening memory difficulties, significant personality changes, and need for assistance with routine daily activities.

- **Stage 7.** Very severe cognitive decline, with individuals unable to respond to their environment, speak recognizably, and, ultimately, control movement.

Diagnosing Alzheimer's Disease[3]

The Alzheimer's Association has developed a list of warning signs that include common symptoms of Alzheimer's. If you or someone close to you exhibits several of the symptoms listed below, you should see a doctor for a complete examination.

- memory loss, especially forgetting names, objects, places, times and dates; inability to recall recently learned information

- difficulty performing everyday tasks; forgetting to maintain personal hygiene
- problems with language; noticeable intellectual decline
- disorientation to time and place; tendency to wander from home or office
- poor or decreased judgment
- problems with abstract thinking; inability to follow simple instructions or stay focused on a task
- misplacing objects or putting things in unusual places
- changes in mood or behavior, especially rapid, unwarranted changes in emotion
- changes in personality, exhibiting extreme confusion, suspicion, fear, or dependence
- loss of initiative, depression, excessive sleeping during daylight hours

If you are concerned that you have symptoms of Alzheimer's disease, you should be thoroughly evaluated by a medical professional. Your doctor will take a current medical and psychological history, assess your neurological status, and evaluate your physical status. You should tell your doctor about any medications or supplements that you are taking. Some medications prescribed for other conditions can cause side effects that mimic some symptoms of Alzheimer's disease. Medical tests might include imaging scans, such as an MRI or CT; laboratory tests, such as blood and urine; neuropsychological tests, such as tests of memory, vision-motor coordination, and language function; and even a psychiatric evaluation to assess emotional factors.

It is important to remember that hormones are closely related to brain health. Hormone levels fluctuate with age, and the importance of consulting with an endocrinologist to assess hormone levels and balance in treating memory deterioration should not be underestimated. Hormones related to memory function include human growth hormone, vasopressin, DHEA, and pregnenolone.

To help your doctor rule out other causes of cognitive impairment, you should be prepared to discuss other possible causes of memory failure. Before settling on a diagnosis of Alzheimer's disease, carefully review the following areas with your doctor.[4]

- **Medication interactions.** Make a list of all substances you are taking, including prescription medications, vitamins, herbal supplements, over-the-counter products such as aspirin or cold medications, smoking-cessation products, weight-loss products, and topical preparations, such as arthritis ointment.

- **Physical conditions.** Ask your doctor to ensure you are not dehydrated. Dehydration can occur from episodes of vomiting or diarrhea or from heat exhaustion. Dehydration is common in older adults, and can interfere with your body's ability to process medications or supplements.
- **Brain traumas.** Report any falls or blows to the head. Falls are common among older adults, and can result in concussions and symptoms similar to those of Alzheimer's.
- **Emotional status.** The symptoms of depression can be remarkably similar to those of dementia. Discuss all possible triggers, such as loss, significant life changes, or side effects of medication—all of which may be underlying causes of depression.
- **Alcohol use.** Consuming too much alcohol or using alcohol with certain medications may cause memory loss.

COMBATING ALZHEIMER'S DISEASE NATURALLY

Scientists have not been able to point to a definitive underlying cause of Alzheimer's disease, nor have they been able to offer a cure for the symptoms. More often than not, conventional medicine recommends drug treatment with a variety of NSAIDs (non-steroidal anti-inflammatory drugs) to stop the progression of Alzheimer's symptoms.

The progressively debilitating disease of Alzheimer's is a serious condition, and it is important to work with your health care provider to find the best treatment for your individual condition. There are safe and natural steps you can take to prevent memory loss, however. Even if you are worried you will develop Alzheimer's disease in later years, if you act now, you can help to prevent memory problems from interfering with your daily life.

Remembering and forgetting things is a perfectly normal part of daily life. But we need not fear that the extreme and progressive cognitive decline that is a symptom of Alzheimer's disease will be an inevitable part of our aging process. There are a number of things we can do to positively impact our brain health and overall mental abilities as we age.

In the Mind Power protocol for impacting Alzheimer's disease that follows, I will tell you how you can make your environment more healthful, exercise your brain to retain memory and mental sharpness, and choose the best foods to help prevent the onset of Alzheimer's disease, or to slow the progression of cognitive decline if you have been diagnosed with this condition.

Lifestyle

In late-stage Alzheimer's there is little that can be done to influence the mood swings, long-term memory loss, verbal outbursts, or delusions that are the hallmarks of the latest stages of the disease. There are several simple ways to prevent the onset of Alzheimer's, however, or to reduce the severity of symptoms if your doctor has diagnosed your memory loss as probable Alzheimer's disease. I have even included some coping strategies to make short-term memory loss less disruptive in your daily routine.

Environment

It is important for your environment to be free of hazardous toxins, particularly heavy metals that can accumulate in the body. High levels of aluminum and mercury are found in the brain cells of Alzheimer's patients. Limit your exposure to cookware, deodorants, antacids, and food additives that contain aluminum. Mercury is found in thermometers, thermostats, and dental amalgams. Chelation therapy, which uses certain amino acids to form strong ionic bonds with the toxic metals in your body, allowing them to be excreted from the system, may be useful in removing toxic metals and other chemicals from your body. Bentonite, a claylike substance that is used in a drink, may be taken at night to draw out toxins from the colon and assist in the detoxification process.

Installing charcoal filters on all water sources used for drinking or cooking can reduce or eliminate harmful toxins that are found in the water from our reservoirs.

Social Activity

Continued community involvement and frequent contact with friends and family may reduce your risk for Alzheimer's disease. In a paper presented at the Alzheimer's Association International Conference on the Prevention of Dementia,[5] Jane Saczynski, Ph.D., of the National Institute on Aging, and colleagues presented data from a longitudinal study, conducted since 1965, that showed that subjects with decreased social activity from mid- to late life had a statistically significant risk of dementia.

Exercise

Physical activity seems to play a role in slowing or preventing the progression of Alzheimer's. A National Institutes of Health news release cites research demonstrating that long-term physical activity increased the learning ability of mice and decreased the level of plaque-forming beta-amyloid protein fragments in their brains.[6] Remaining physically active throughout our lifetimes offers immeasurable benefits to both body and brain. Physical activity does not have to be rigorous. Walking, dancing, or practicing yoga all help safeguard our brains against the type of cognitive decline that is a symptom of Alzheimer's disease.

Memory Skills and Brain Boosters

In addition to an active body, it is important to have an active mind. A study published in the *New England Journal of Medicine* supports the theory that mentally demanding activities can help stave off dementia.[7] The study involved 469 people aged seventy-five and older. Those participants who read, played games of strategy, such as checkers, backgammon or chess, played musical instruments, or danced at least twice a week were significantly less likely to develop dementia. Those who did crossword puzzles four times a week were also found to have a significantly lowered risk. It seems clear that participating in mentally stimulating hobbies and being willing to learn new information and challenge our brains on an ongoing basis provide important benefits in preventing the symptoms of Alzheimer's disease.

Coping Strategies

If you or someone close to you has been diagnosed as being in the early stages of Alzheimer's, there are some strategies for coping with the symptoms of memory loss that may be the first hallmarks of this disease. These coping strategies will help relieve the stress and tension that arise from memory problems, and can help lessen the impact of such problems on day-to-day life. Remember, in addition to practicing the strategies outlined below, you should make the lifestyle and nutritional changes I recommend in this chapter to slow or reverse the progression of these early symptoms.

- Establish a regular routine in familiar surroundings.
- Make mental associations, such as using landmarks, to help you find things.
- Repeat names when you meet people.
- Put important items, such as your keys, in the same place every time.
- Label or color-code doors and exits to keep from getting disoriented.
- Draw a map for simple routes. Write down directions.
- Make lists, use a calendar, and keep notes of important dates and financial matters.
- Set realistic daily goals.
- Keep track of when medicines are taken; use a chart or special pill box to stay current.
- Tell your doctor about all medications or supplements you are taking.
- Keep a list of important names and numbers near the telephone.
- Stay in frequent contact with family and friends.

Nutrition

What can be difficult in promoting proper nutrition as we age is the fact that our bodies may become less efficient in absorbing and utilizing key nutrients. Therefore, it is important that every bit of food you eat has the maximum positive impact on your mental health.

Foods and Alzheimer's Disease

As research into the causes of Alzheimer's continues, researchers are concluding that there may be ways in which we can limit our risk of developing Alzheimer's disease. What these researchers are beginning to say now is something that I have said over and over again: deficiencies of essential nutrients can lead to a variety of health problems and leave us vulnerable to serious conditions such as Alzheimer's. The good news is that it is never too early to start good nutritional habits that will help to protect the brain over a lifetime. And it is never too late to benefit from good nutritional habits.

Most Americans today eat foods that are overprocessed and far from their natural state. These processed foods have been stripped of vital nutrients and filled with additives, processed sugars, and trans fats.

In addition to nutrients lost through poor diet, nutritional deficiencies may simply increase as we age. To help ensure that our bodies get the nutrients we need, we must make an effort to eat foods in their natural state. For

people suffering from Alzheimer's it is vitally important to purchase organic foods whenever possible, since these foods are more likely to have
trace minerals like chromium, magnesium, selenium, and zinc, which are
vital to the brain's health.

Various studies support the efficacy of antioxidants as a method of preventing or reversing cognitive decline. Vitamins E and C are proven free
radical fighters and are readily available in foods like citrus fruits and juices,
dark green, leafy vegetables, nuts, and sunflower seeds. The B vitamins,
which play an important role in fighting the symptoms of Alzheimer's disease, are found in fish, eggs, beans, and animal proteins. Trace minerals like
zinc, magnesium, and potassium are easy to add to our diets by using whole
grains, nuts, dried beans, bananas, and milk.

Essential fatty acids (EFAs) such as omega-3 and omega-6 fats, which
are found in cold-water fish like salmon, mackerel, sardines, and herring, as
well as in flax oil, walnuts, and oysters, have significant anti-inflammatory
properties and may be important in preventing Alzheimer's. It has been
suggested that a dietary deficiency in fatty acids may be a risk factor for
Alzheimer's.[8] Other studies have looked at the use of EFAs in impacting
Alzheimer's and found them to be beneficial.[9]

Recipes

The recipes at the end of this book are intended to help you get started on a
healthy eating plan that will provide optimum mental health benefits. Each
dish focuses on foods rich in vitamins and nutrients beneficial to our brains.
Eating right does not have to involve a huge effort. Prepare healthy dishes in
larger quantities and store them for use throughout the week. In the list below are my recommendations for easy-to-prepare meals full of nutrients
proven to help prevent and reduce the symptoms of Alzheimer's disease.

Antioxidant Punch, page 252
Blueberry and Pear Macadamia Nut Shake, page 253
Brain Power, page 254
Carrot, Pineapple, and Strawberry Juice, page 254
Everglades Punch, page 258
Flax Cruncher, page 259
Free Radical Delight, page 259
Nuts and Seeds, page 262
Velvety Pecan Milk, page 265

Four Bean Salad, page 266
Mixed Sprout, Bean, and Nut Salad, page 271
Black Bean Soup, page 275
Cream of Barley, page 281
Nutty Oatmeal, page 281
Gary's Veggieball Stew, page 284
Indonesian Kale, page 286
Pasta Fagioli, page 288
Sweet Kidney Bean Mash, page 290
Heavenly Roasted Nuts, page 296

Supplements

Even with a diet rich in recommended vitamins and minerals, your body may not efficiently absorb and process these necessary nutrients. As you grow older, your appetite may decrease, and you may find that you are unable to consistently take in the recommended amounts of food nutrients. It may be that getting these nutrients in supplement form is the most efficient way for you to enhance your healthy diet. However, supplements are not intended to replace healthy food choices.

Of course, before you begin any new health program, you should get a comprehensive, full-body evaluation performed by a qualified health care practitioner. A proper health and medical evaluation should evaluate your blood chemistry to assess your blood markers, your metabolic rate, and your blood pressure for indicators of cardiovascular, hormonal, or other imbalances or danger signs. If you are taking medications of any sort, for Alzheimer's disease or any other condition, you need to inform your doctor of any supplements you are considering adding to your daily diet, as some may interact with prescription medications and cause adverse effects. You should speak to your doctor before adding any of these supplements to your daily regimen.

Vitamins and Minerals

Certain vitamins and minerals are very important in fighting the symptoms of Alzheimer's disease.

MAGNESIUM Magnesium is well known for its calming properties in persons with anxiety symptoms, but proper amounts of magnesium are generally lacking in the average American diet. Individuals who use oral contraceptives or diuretics, and who overuse laxatives, are at risk of magnesium deficiency. Magnesium also assists in impacting circulatory problems. For impacting the symptoms of Alzheimer's, I recommend a daily supplement of 500–1,000 mg of magnesium, taken in two equal doses on an empty stomach.

POTASSIUM Potassium is one of the most abundant minerals in the human body. Most of the time supplementation with potassium is unnecessary, because it is so readily available in our diet in such foods as bananas, orange juice, and potatoes. Potassium is depleted from our bodies in times of stress, thus upsetting the delicate balance of neurotransmitter communication in our brains. For this reason, potassium supplements may be useful in impacting Alzheimer's. Potassium can interact with some drugs, so if you are taking prescription medications, consult with your doctor before taking potassium supplements. If potassium is safe for you, I recommend a daily supplement of 500 mg.

VITAMIN B COMPLEX It is important that your daily vitamin B complex contain sufficient amounts of both vitamin B_9 and B_{12}, as deficiencies in these vitamins can develop as we age, and these deficiencies can contribute to the symptoms of Alzheimer's disease. If your doctor has determined you are deficient in B vitamins, you may want to ask about receiving intravenous or injected supplements of vitamin B complex to combat symptoms of Alzheimer's.

VITAMIN C Vitamin C may help delay the onset of Alzheimer's and slow the progression of symptoms. For best impact on the symptoms of Alzheimer's disease, I recommend increasing your daily supplement from 500–1,000 mg to 3,000 mg, taken in three divided doses. Do not exceed a daily supplement of 3,000 mg.

VITAMIN E Vitamin E has beneficial antioxidant properties, and treatment with high doses has shown initial promise in slowing the progression of symptoms in individuals with moderately severe Alzheimer's.[10] Because vitamin E has anticoagulant properties, and high doses may be associated with the risk of bleeding and interaction with anticoagulants and other medications often taken by elderly people, you should discuss high-dose vitamin E supplementation with your doctor. If you are not at risk, I recommend increasing your daily supplement of vitamin E from 400 IU to 800 IU, taken in two divided doses. Do not exceed a daily supplement of 800 IU.

ZINC Many people who suffer from dementia have deficiencies in zinc. I recommend a daily supplement of 30 mg.

Smart Drugs and Nutrients

A number of other naturally occurring nutrients have a beneficial impact on the symptoms of Alzheimer's disease.

ACETYL-L-CARNITINE (ACL) This versatile nutrient is able to permeate the blood-brain barrier to stimulate and fortify the brain's nerve cells. Acetyl-L-carnitine is a type of carnitine produced naturally in the brain. It can aid in directing fatty acids to the cell mitochondria, assisting in the creation of new cell energy. A powerful antioxidant, acetyl-L-carnitine also supplements the neurotransmitter acetylcholine. For best impact on Alzheimer's symptoms, I recommend increasing your daily supplement from 2,000 mg to 3,000 mg, taken in three equal doses. Do not exceed a daily supplement of 3,000 mg.

DMAE (DIMETHYLAMINOETHANOL) This nutrient, found in sardines, is a powerful brain stimulant that increases acetylcholine—a neurotransmitter essential for short-term memory function and concentration. Some side effects associated with DMAE in Alzheimer's patients include drowsiness, high blood pressure, and increased confusion. If you experience these symptoms, stop taking the supplement for a few days, then return to your lower daily dose. I recommend increasing your daily supplement from 150 mg to 300 mg, taken in two equal doses with meals. Do not exceed a daily supplement of 300 mg.

L-GLUTAMINE Glutamine is one of the most abundant nonessential amino acids in the bloodstream. It is produced in the muscles and is able to pass freely through the blood-brain barrier. Once in the brain, it is converted into glutamic acid and increases GABA, a neurotransmitter essential for proper mental function. There are two types of glutamine supplements: D-glutamine and L-glutamine. L-glutamine is the form that more closely mimics the glutamine in the body. To impact the symptoms of Alzheimer's disease, I recommend supplementing with 500 mg, taken three times daily.

MELATONIN Melatonin is a hormone manufactured by the pineal gland in the brain. It is released into the bloodstream, and is involved in synchronizing the body's hormone secretions and setting daily biorhythms. It is one of the body's most potent antioxidants. To stabilize the sleeping cycle for Alzheimer's patients, I recommend supplementing with 300 mcg to 1 mg, taken nightly a half hour before bed.

NAC (N-ACETYLCYSTEINE) This amino acid protects the brain from damaging free radicals by boosting quantities of glutathione, one of the body's most powerful antioxidants. I recommend a supplement of 500 mg, taken three times daily.

NADH (NICOTINAMIDE ADENINE DINUCLEOTIDE) An enzyme that helps improve neurotransmitter function, NADH is present in all living cells and plays a critical role in energy production. It helps prevent cellular degeneration, and may increase concentration and memory capacity. I recommend a supplement of 2.5 mg, taken twice a day for two or three days of the week.

PS (PHOSPHATIDYLSERINE) PS helps the brain use fuel more efficiently. By boosting neuronal metabolism and stimulating production of acetylcholine, PS may be able to improve the condition of patients in cognitive decline. Studies have revealed that supplementing with phosphatidylserine slows down—and even reverses—declining memory and concentration, or age-related cognitive impairment in middle-aged and elderly subjects.[11]

As we grow older, aging slows the body's manufacturing of phosphatidylserine to levels that are detrimental to our functioning at our full mental capacity. For impact on memory loss, I recommend increasing your daily supplement from 300 mg to 400 mg. Do not exceed a daily supplement of 400 mg.

SAME (S-ADENOSYLMETHIONINE) SAMe (pronounced "sammy") has long been prescribed by European doctors as a treatment for depression. SAMe promotes cell growth and repair, and maintains levels of glutathione, a major antioxidant that protects against free radicals and reduces homocysteine levels. Alzheimer patients have extremely low levels of SAMe in their brains. SAMe should not be taken if you are taking MAO inhibitor antidepressants. You should consult with your doctor before taking SAMe if you suffer from severe depression or bipolar disorder. If SAMe is safe for you to use, I recommend a daily supplement of 400–1,600 mg daily taken in four equal doses.

Mind Power Chart of Additional Supplements for Impacting Alzheimer's Disease

The following chart summarizes the supplements I recommend adding to the protocol for overall brain health from Chapter 2. In some cases I will recommend increasing the dose of a vitamin or supplement to specifically impact Alzheimer's disease. In these cases, you should increase the daily dosage from Chapter 2 to the level recommended for this specific condition.

This protocol is designed for individuals who suffer from, or are specifically concerned about, Alzheimer's disease. If you are concerned about additional brain conditions discussed in other chapters, consult with a health professional about how you can safely impact multiple conditions.

If you are taking medications—whether prescription or over-the-counter—or have any food restrictions, consult with your doctor before beginning any supplement program. Your health care provider should always be up-to-date on all vitamins, supplements, and herbal or homeopathic remedies you are taking. Supplement overdoses are rare, but possible, and certain combinations may affect individuals adversely.

Supplement	Dosage	Cautions
acetyl-L-carnitine (ACL)	I recommend increasing your daily supplement from 2,000 mg to 3,000 mg, taken in three equal doses. Do not exceed a daily supplement of 3,000 mg.	
DMAE (dimethyl-aminoethanol)	Increase daily dosage from 150 mg to 300 mg, taken in	Do not take DMAE if you have epilepsy, a history of

Supplement	Dosage	Cautions
DMAE (dimethyl–aminoethanol) (*cont.*)	two equal doses with meals. Do not exceed a daily supplement of 300 mg.	convulsions, or bipolar disorder. If you have kidney or liver disease, consult with your doctor before taking DMAE. Some side effects associated with DMAE in Alzheimer's patients include drowsiness, high blood pressure, and increased confusion. If you experience these symptoms, stop taking the supplement for a few days, then return to your lower daily dose.
intravenous vitamin B complex	Discuss with your health care provider whether you might benefit from injected vitamin B.	
L–glutamine	500 mg taken three times daily	
magnesium	500–1,000 mg in two equal doses	Take on an empty stomach. If loose stools occur, decrease dosage. May take six weeks or more for effects to be felt.
melatonin	300 mcg–1 mg at night a half hour before bed	Tolerance may develop with regular use. Long-term effects of nightly use are unknown.
NAC (N-acetylcysteine)	500 mg three times daily	Regular supplementation of NAC increases urinary output of copper. If supplementing with NAC for an extended period, add 2 mg of copper and 30 mg of zinc to your daily supplement regimen.

continued . . .

Supplement	Dosage	Cautions
NADH (nicotinamide adenine dinucleotide, or coenzyme Q1)	2.5 mg twice daily, two or three times per week	High doses (10 mg per day or more) may cause nervousness, anxiety, and insomnia.
PS (phos-phatidylserine)	Increase daily dosage from 300 mg to 400 mg. Do not exceed a daily supplement of 400 mg.	
potassium	500 mg daily	Do not take potassium supplements if you are taking medications for high blood pressure or heart disease, or if you have a kidney disorder. Consuming foods rich in potassium is okay. Do not exceed 3.5 grams daily without consulting your doctor.
SAMe (S–adenosyl-methionine)	Dosage range of 400–1,600 mg	Raise the dose gradually from 200 mg twice a day to 400 mg twice a day, to 400 mg three times a day, to 400 mg four times a day, over a period of twenty days.
vitamin C	Increase daily dosage from 500–1,000 mg to 3,000 mg, taken in three divided doses. Do not exceed a daily supplement of 3,000 mg.	
vitamin E	Increase daily dosage from 400 IU to 800 IU, taken in two divided doses. Do not exceed a daily supplement of 800 IU.	Vitamin E may cause increased risk of bleeding, and may have adverse inter-actions with anticoagulants or other medications. Consult with your doctor

Supplement	Dosage	Cautions
vitamin E (*cont.*)		before beginning high-dose supplementation with vitamin E.
zinc	Up to 30 mg daily	Large doses (50 mg or more) can interfere with the body's absorption of essential minerals, impair blood cell function, and depress the immune system.

Alternative Health Remedies

When suffering from a specific condition like Alzheimer's disease, we can also try some natural treatment options that are considered "alternatives" to traditional medicine. While a healthful lifestyle and the proper nutritional and supplement plan are vital to winning the battle against the symptoms of Alzheimer's, there are some other targeted remedies that might help, too.

Herbal Remedies

Some herbal extracts and homeopathic treatments have properties similar to conventional medications, but are gentler and may lack the drugs' side effects. Always inform your medical practitioner of any herbal remedies you may be taking.

- **Butcher's broom** is an herb that promotes clearer focus and enhanced memory. I recommend a daily supplement of 850 mg taken in two equal doses.
- *Bacopa monnieri* is a potent antioxidant that has been used in Ayurvedic medicine for centuries as a brain tonic to enhance memory, learning, development, and concentration. I recommend a daily supplement of 200–400 mg taken in two equal doses.
- **Ginkgo biloba** is an herbal extract derived from the ginkgo biloba tree. It is commonly used in Europe to help fight Alzheimer's disease. Ginkgo biloba is a potent antioxidant that may be beneficial in

impacting dementia-related symptoms. By improving circulation to the central nervous system, ginkgo biloba may help to stabilize abnormal neurotransmitter communication in the brain. In a study conducted at the New York Institute for Medical Research, researchers found that almost one-third of Alzheimer's patients taking ginkgo supplements showed improvements in cognitive function during a double-blind, placebo-controlled clinical study.[12] Ginkgo can act as an anticoagulant, and individuals taking anticoagulant and antithrombotic drugs like ASA, anti-inflammatories, and warfarin or Coumadin should consult with their doctor before taking ginkgo. If ginkgo is safe for you to take, for prevention of Alzheimer's disease, I recommend a daily supplement of 120 mg taken in two equal doses. For those suffering from more advanced stages of the disease, I recommend increasing your daily dose to 240 mg, spread out over three daily doses.

- **KUT** (*Kami-Untan-To*) is a Japanese herbal medicine that has been used for centuries in Japan to combat neuropsychiatric problems. In animal studies KUT has been shown to increase choline acetyltransferase levels and nerve growth factor.[13] Later studies showed that KUT may be beneficial as an interventional strategy to fight Alzheimer's disease by slowing cognitive decline.[14] KUT is a blend of thirteen different herbs and should be taken as directed by the manufacturer.

- **Huperzine A** is a compound isolated from a Chinese herb called *Hyperzia serrata*. It increases acetylcholine activity in the cortex and hippocampus sections of the brain, and aids in improving memory as well as cognitive and behavioral functions. In a double-blind, placebo-controlled study conducted in China, 103 individuals with Alzheimer's disease received either huperzine A or a placebo twice daily for eight weeks. About 60 percent of the participants treated with huperzine A showed significant improvements in memory, thinking, and behavioral functions, compared to 36 percent of the placebo-treated subjects.[15] For an impact on Alzheimer's symptoms, I recommend taking a daily supplement of 100–200 mcg in two equal doses.

- **St. John's wort** (*Hypericum*) is very popular in Europe, so much so that it is actually covered by German health insurance as a prescription drug. I recommend taking a daily supplement of 300 mg twice per day.

- **Vinpocetine** is a derivative of an extract taken from the periwinkle shrub. It enhances circulation to the brain, and may prevent or improve mild cognitive impairment. I recommend taking 10 mg twice daily with meals.

Homeopathic Remedies

The following remedies may be used to impact the symptoms of Alzheimer's. When dealing with a chronic condition, homeopathic remedies must be used in conjunction with other therapies, as prescribed by a qualified health professional. Consult with your health care provider before taking any homeopathic remedy, and follow their recommendation for the appropriate dosage. Always inform your medical practitioner of any homeopathic remedies you may be taking.

- *Alumina* is indicated for dealing with great weakness or loss of memory in cases where consciousness of personal identity is confused.
- *Anacardium* is used for absentmindedness; memory for names is most affected.
- *Calcarea* may help when the person is elderly, wandering, and finds words difficult to remember.
- **Sulphur** can be used when there is difficulty remembering words or names.

Aromatherapy

Essential oils can be used in baths or inhaled to provide an energizing or soothing effect. Do not apply essential oils directly to the skin; they must be mixed with carrier oils. Experiment with various scents to see which help to alleviate the symptoms of Alzheimer's and increase mental clarity.

- bergamot
- clove
- frankincense
- lavender
- lemon balm

SUMMARY

Contrary to mainstream medical belief, there are safe, natural, and nontoxic treatments for the symptoms of Alzheimer's disease. Research has demonstrated how these remedies can aid in preventing the onset of Alzheimer's or alleviating symptoms that have developed. In the past, Alzheimer's disease was considered an uncontrollable force that caused elderly patients to wither away and die. Taking action now can prevent our elder years from being characterized by cognitive degeneration and a rapid decline in health and ability.

CHAPTER 9

HEADACHES

Virtually everyone gets headaches, but not all headaches are the same. Recurring—or chronic—headaches, particularly migraine headaches, are one of the primary reasons people visit doctors. People who suffer from headache also seek relief from hypnotists, chiropractors, and alternative health practitioners. Headaches, while not considered a disease, can indicate a serious underlying condition.

The good news is that as we grow older, our tendency to suffer from headaches decreases. Chronic headache onset is unusual in people older than fifty. Even migraines may lessen or disappear with age. The more concerning news is that headaches in older individuals can be a symptom of a more serious underlying illness.

Even if there is no illness causing your headaches, they can still be debilitating. Headaches can range from the pressure and pain of a tension headache to the pain of a migraine, which may be so severe it prevents you from performing even the simplest task. According to MAGNUM, the Migraine Awareness Group: A National Understanding for Migraineurs, approximately 32 million people in the United States today suffer from migraine headaches.

In this chapter we'll look at types of headaches and their probable causes, including drug interactions or chemical changes in the brain. I'll discuss some important changes you can make in your lifestyle and diet to help prevent the onset of headaches. And I'll tell you what kinds of alternative treatments and remedies may provide you with relief from chronic headaches or migraines.

UNDERSTANDING HEADACHES

Despite the number of trips to a doctor and missed workdays caused by severe headaches, they are not considered a disease. They can be symptoms of an illness, such as a viral or bacterial infection, allergies, or sinus infections. Fever may also cause headaches. Headaches can also be caused by factors such as hunger, stress, dehydration, drugs, sleep problems, head injuries, or certain foods.

Many doctors believe migraines are the result of a chemical or electrical problem in the brain. During a migraine, the cerebral blood vessels constrict tightly, and then quickly expand. Many believe that the nervous system, in response to a trigger—such as stress—generates spasms in the nerve-rich arteries in the base of the skull. These spasms squeeze many of the arteries that supply blood to the brain, reducing the flow of oxygen-rich blood. In response to the lack of oxygen, cerebral arteries in the brain dilate, triggering the release of neurotransmitters that elicit inflammation and pain responses.

In order to prevent and impact occurrences of headache, it is important to understand what type of headache you may be suffering from. In the section that follows, we'll look at types of headaches that are common at any age.

Types of Headaches

In the discussion of types, diagnosis, and ways to impact headaches that follows, I will briefly discuss several types of headache, but will focus primarily on tension headaches—the most common type of headache—and migraine headaches—the most severe type of headache. Both have commonly identified triggers and generally exhibit positive responses to changes in nutrition and lifestyle.

Hypnic Headaches

This newly described type of headache that occurs in elderly patients is easy to recognize. Hypnic headaches—so called because they arise out of sleep—present as bilateral pain that lasts for thirty to sixty minutes, awakening patients from sleep one or two times each night. Hypnic headaches occur primarily in individuals over age sixty-five and respond well to treatment with medication (most often lithium, taken at bedtime).

Cluster Headaches

Cluster headaches come in groups. They can last for extended periods of time—for days, weeks, or even months. Sufferers usually experience one or more headaches per day. Each headache may be relatively brief, lasting for thirty to ninety minutes, and may escalate in intensity during that time. In general, cluster headaches affect one side of the head, and the pain is centralized in the eye area on the affected side.

Exertion Headaches

Exertion headaches are connected to physical activities like exercise, sex, laughing, and coughing. They generally occur during or just after the activity. In and of themselves they are not dangerous, but frequent exertion headaches may indicate an underlying physical state conducive to stroke or another serious condition.

Organic Headaches

Headaches that are the symptoms of a serious underlying physical condition, such as high blood pressure or brain tumors, are considered organic headaches. In addition to the headache pain, the sufferer may have fever, confusion, and/or trouble speaking or moving. The pain tends to grow worse, either increasing with each headache or striking more frequently.

Migraine Headaches

Migraines are less common in individuals over the age of fifty, but may first occur in our later years. Migraine headaches are characterized by severe, throbbing pain—often on one side of the head, though the entire head may be involved—and may be accompanied by light-headedness and nausea and/or vomiting. Sufferers of migraines may be sensitive to sound, light, and smells. The pain from a migraine can last from a few hours to a few days.

Classic migraines strike on one side of the head and are preceded by warning signs called auras, which are commonly experienced as spots of light or changes in vision, although visual, auditory, and olfactory hallucinations can also rarely occur. These auras precede the migraine attack by ten to thirty minutes.

A migraine attack can leave the sufferer listless, exhausted, and vulnerable to other mental or physical conditions.

Tension Headaches

Tension headaches are characterized by a dull, aching pain that radiates throughout the entire head. Some sufferers describe the feeling as having a tight band wrapped around their head. Tension headaches can start in the shoulders and neck and move upward to the back of the head. Stress, arguments, repressed anger, poor posture, depression, social problems, or major life changes can induce tension headaches. Tension headaches may also be a symptom of depression, especially in the elderly who have experienced a potentially traumatic or stressful event, such as retirement, forced relocation, reduced mobility or independence, or a serious illness.

Diagnosing Headaches

Chronic headaches, or headaches that change in character or suddenly develop in an older person, should be carefully evaluated. They may be the result of a drug interaction or carbon monoxide poisoning. Headaches may also be the symptom of a more serious condition, such as giant cell arteritis (a condition of the arteries of the optic nerves that can result in blindness), brain tumors, spinal degeneration, or lung disease, or even a warning sign of stroke. Determining if you are suffering from tension headaches and migraine headaches can let you take steps to prevent future occurrences. Both of these types of headache also respond well to both conventional and alternative treatments.

Keeping a daily journal of headache occurrences may help you and your doctor to understand what is causing your headaches. I counsel migraine sufferers in my support groups to keep a detailed record of all medications and supplements they are taking, as well as all food and drink they consume. In addition to these daily accounts, I encourage them to record the frequency, location, duration, and timing of the headaches, as well as the type of pain and any tangential symptoms (such as nausea or vision disturbances) that accompany or precede the headache. Because a combination of triggers may be responsible for the occurrence of chronic headache, a journal such as the one I've described can reveal areas in lifestyle and nutrition where you need to make changes.

Women tend to suffer more from migraine, and hormones may play a role. Some women suffer from migraines during their menstrual period. Other migraine sufferers may find that the headaches stop when they are pregnant. Women who take oral contraceptives may also be susceptible to migraine.

A number of medications, many of which are commonly prescribed as we grow older, may cause headaches. Your doctor may ask if you are taking any over-the-counter medications. He may also want to know if you take or have changed your dosage of any of the following commonly prescribed medications: cardiovascular drugs, such as vasodilator or nitroglycerin; antiarrhythmia drugs; blood pressure medications; Parkinson's drugs, such as L-dopa; sedatives; stimulants, including caffeine; NSAIDs (non-steroidal anti-inflammatory drugs); some analgesics; histamine blockers, such as Tagamet or Zantac; bronchodilators; antibiotics, especially trimethoprim-sulfamethoxazole (Bactrim, Septa).

If you are worried about your headaches, or if they are disruptive to your daily functioning, you should consult with your health care provider. If your headaches follow a recent head injury, are associated with seizures, are so severe they prevent you from doing activities you want to do, wake you from sleep, cause blurred vision, eyespots or other visual changes, or are associated with fever, vomiting, stiff neck, or tooth, jaw, or sinus pain, you should consult with your doctor immediately.

Tension and migraine are the most commonly diagnosed chronic headache conditions, and I discuss the symptoms of each in more detail below.

Symptoms of Tension Headaches

Tension headaches may happen daily or episodically. Episodic occurrences are usually the result of stressful events. This type of headache is generally of moderate intensity and responds well to nonprescription drugs or alternative treatment. Chronic tension headache usually occurs daily, and is associated with contracted muscles of the neck and scalp. Other symptoms of tension headaches are:

- feeling of pressure or tightness
- pain in the front of the head or eye area
- mild to moderate intensity
- duration of thirty minutes up to seven days
- no nausea or vomiting
- sensitivity to sound or light
- minimum of ten previous episodes; fewer than 180 days per year with headache
- occurs acutely when you are under emotional distress or intense worry

- may cause insomnia
- often occurs upon waking, or shortly thereafter
- not aggravated by physical activity

Symptoms of Migraine Headaches

Migraine headaches can be caused by heredity or by specific triggers or by a combination of triggers. The pain may be felt in the whole head, or on just one side. Some people experience an "aura" before a migraine attack, but most people do not have warning of when a migraine will strike unless they are aware of their own specific triggers for this type of headache. Symptoms of a migraine include:

- predictive aura, such as blind spots, flashing lights, wavy or tunnel vision
- visual, auditory, or olfactory hallucination (rare)
- physical weakness or exhaustion
- throbbing pain
- duration of four to seventy-two hours
- nausea
- vomiting
- sensitivity to light or sound
- light-headedness
- neurological abnormalities, such as confusion, seizures, or impairment of consciousness
- ocular muscle paralysis (rare)
- aphasia (rare)

COMBATING HEADACHES NATURALLY

Although the onset of debilitating headaches becomes less common as we grow older, those individuals who are prone to tension headaches or migraines may continue to experience them as they age. Taking steps to prevent these headaches at any age will lessen the chances of headaches, becoming a factor in your brain health as you grow older. As I pointed out above, however, a medical professional should evaluate any sudden onset of headache in an elderly person to rule out drug interactions, an underlying medical condition, or the unusual syndrome of hypnic headaches.

In the Mind Power protocol for impacting headaches that follows, I'll suggest ways to use alternative therapies and nutritional strategies to prevent severe and debilitating headaches at any age.

Lifestyle

Attention to specific areas of your lifestyle can be crucial in preventing headache. Any behavior that promotes a healthful lifestyle, such as regular sleeping schedules, managing stress, practicing relaxation techniques, and staying physically fit, can reduce the frequency and intensity of both tension and migraine headaches. When the pain is in your brain, the importance of the mind/body connection becomes paramount.

Exercise

Studies have shown that moderate exercise can release endorphins and natural cortisol, which act to elevate mood and reduce stress. Aerobic exercise, such as dancing, walking, biking, or swimming, can help reduce the frequency of tension headaches. Gentle exercises, such as stretching, yoga, or even walking, can reduce discomfort while releasing stress. Exercise is also beneficial in normalizing sleep patterns and enhancing self-confidence. To ensure that you stay on a regular exercise regimen, I suggest that you choose a pleasurable activity and stick with it.

Meditation

Meditation acts to calm the mind and relieve stress. Twenty minutes, twice a day, of mindful meditation is recommended to prevent and reduce tension and stress. Engaging in breathing exercises and being generally aware of your breathing patterns throughout the day can be beneficial in eliminating headaches. Focusing on the positive aspects of life and nurturing an optimistic outlook will reduce the effects of stress on the body and aid in coping with headaches.

Posture

It may sound simple—and it is. Standing and sitting correctly can keep your muscles from tensing and triggering a tension headache. Good posture supports and protects all of your body, allowing you to move efficiently and with less fatigue. When standing, make sure your weight is evenly distributed on both feet, hold your shoulders back, and tuck in your chin. Pull in your abdomen and buttocks. When sitting, make sure your thighs are parallel to the ground and your head is not slumped forward. Try to avoid standing or sitting in one position for long periods of time. Take frequent breaks to move around and stretch. Make sure your shoes fit correctly, and do not make a habit of wearing high heels regularly.

Nutrition

What can be difficult in promoting proper nutrition as we age is the fact that our bodies may become less efficient in absorbing and utilizing key nutrients. Therefore, it is important that every bit of food you eat has the maximum positive impact on your mental health.

Foods and Headaches

Studies indicate that a poor diet may be a significant factor in triggering headaches, particularly migraines. To prevent and impact migraine headaches, I recommend some very specific dietary guidelines.

One of the most important steps is the elimination of caffeine from your diet. Caffeine and caffeinelike substances found in coffee, tea, and many soft drinks can cause symptoms of anxiety, such as nervousness, fear, heart palpitations, nausea, restlessness, and tremors. Caffeine overstimulates the adrenal system and can deplete your body of important B-complex and C vitamins. It can cause stress and anxiety reactions in users. One study shows that patients with anxiety experienced a degree of anxiety that directly correlated with their consumption of caffeine. Even more astonishing, this report suggested that the persons most at risk for suffering from anxiety effects have a heightened sensitivity to the effects of just one cup of coffee.[1]

Ironically, the process of eliminating caffeine from your diet may cause a withdrawal headache, as your body compensates for the lack of caffeine by producing more adenosine, a neurotransmitter that helps to regulate the diameter of the arteries in your head. As adenosine levels increase, your arteries dilate, and the excessive blood flow can then cause a throbbing headache. Once your body begins to regulate adenosine levels, however, the withdrawal headache will cease and you should remain headache-free.

Hypoglycemia (lowered blood glucose levels) is also directly correlated to headache and its related symptoms. To compensate for lowered glucose levels, your body releases insulin, a hormone that encourages glucose to move from the bloodstream into the cells. A sudden drop in blood sugar may cause the arteries in your brain to constrict, contributing to high blood pressure and headache. Maintaining proper blood sugar levels by avoiding refined carbohydrates is essential to controlling headaches.

Another common trigger for headaches is sensitivity to certain chemicals in foods. These chemicals include MSG (monosodium glutamate), a common flavor enhancer found in many processed foods; artificial sweeteners found in diet foods and diet soft drinks; nitrites, preservatives found in processed meats and some cheeses; and amines, a common compound found in a wide range of foods, including spinach, tomato, potato, small whole fish, tuna, liver, dark chocolate, and alcohol.

Phenols, a serotonin-depleting compound found in red wine, may also trigger migraine. Of course, drinking too much alcohol may trigger not only migraine headache, but may cause the headache of a hangover, which is due largely to dehydration.

Headache sufferers should be conscious of the foods they eat. Choose organic, chemical-free foods and eat regular meals to avoid hypoglycemic reactions. Keep a food journal that lets you see if there are food-related patterns to your headaches. When a headache occurs, review the foods you ate in the seventy-two hours prior to its onset to see if you can identify any trends. If you suspect a particular food may cause headaches, try eating that specific food for a week and see if it triggers a headache. If it does, avoid it in the future.

Recipes

The recipes at the end of this book are intended to help you get started on a healthy eating plan that will provide optimum mental health benefits. Each dish focuses on foods rich in vitamins and nutrients beneficial to our brains. Eating right does not have to involve a huge effort. Prepare healthy dishes in larger quantities and store them for use throughout the week. In the list below are my recommendations for easy-to-prepare meals full of nutrients proven to help prevent headache.

Supplements

Even with a diet rich in recommended vitamins and minerals, your body may not efficiently absorb and process these necessary nutrients. As you grow older, your appetite may decrease, and you may find that you are unable to consistently take in the recommended amounts of food nutrients. It may be that getting these nutrients in supplement form is the most efficient way for you to enhance your healthy diet. However, supplements are not intended to replace healthy food choices.

Of course, before you begin any new health program, you should get a comprehensive, full-body evaluation performed by a qualified health care practitioner. A proper health and medical evaluation should evaluate your blood chemistry to assess your blood markers, your metabolic rate, and your blood pressure for indicators of cardiovascular, hormonal, or other imbalances or danger signs. If you are taking medications of any sort, for headaches or any other condition, you need to inform your doctor of any supplements you are considering adding to your daily diet, as some may interact with prescription medications and cause adverse effects. You should speak to your doctor before adding any of these supplements to your daily regimen.

Vitamins and Minerals

Certain vitamins and minerals are very important in the prevention of headache.

MAGNESIUM About half of the people who suffer migraines are deficient in the free and active form of magnesium called ionized magnesium.[2] Magnesium's role in fighting migraine is undeniable. It has the ability to relax muscles, including those that encircle the arteries. Magnesium also affects serotonin receptors.

A double-blind study conducted to examine the effectiveness of magnesium on migraines showed that when given to patients on a daily basis, it reduced migraine attacks by 42 percent after nine weeks.[3] If you suffer from migraines, I recommend a daily supplement of 1,000 mg of free-form magnesium from citrate. Be sure you are taking a daily B-complex vitamin along with the magnesium, as vitamin B_3 plays an important role in aiding the absorption of magnesium.

VITAMIN B_2 (RIBOFLAVIN) Vitamin B_2 is important in mitochondrial energy production. In individuals suffering from migraine, mitochondrial energy production may be low. To optimize this cellular energy production, I recommend increasing your daily supplement from 50 mg to 150 mg. Do not exceed a daily supplement of 150 mg.

VITAMIN B_3 (NIACIN) Vitamin B_3 may aid in preventing migraine headaches by opening constricted arteries and increasing blood flow. At the onset of a migraine aura, I recommend taking a supplement of 100–150 mg of vitamin B_3.

Smart Drugs and Nutrients

Other naturally occurring nutrients may have beneficial impacts on headaches.

5-HTP (5-HYDROXYTRYPTOPHAN) 5-HTP is a form of the amino acid tryptophan that the body converts into serotonin, and can be effective in preventing migraines. I recommend 50–100 mg taken three times daily.

MELATONIN Research has shown that migraine sufferers are low in melatonin,[4] a hormone produced by the pineal gland to aid in sleep and setting our circadian rhythms. Melatonin also has an anti-inflammatory effect and is a powerful antioxidant. To prevent migraines, I recommend a supplement of 300 mcg–1 mg taken a half hour before bed, two to three nights per week.

Mind Power Chart of Additional Supplements for Impacting Headache

The following chart summarizes the supplements I recommend adding to the protocol for overall brain health from Chapter 2. In some cases I will recommend increasing the dose of a particular vitamin or supplement to specifically impact headache. In these cases, you should increase the daily dosage from Chapter 2 to the level recommended for this specific condition.

This protocol is designed for individuals who suffer from, or are specifically concerned about, headache. If you are concerned about additional brain conditions discussed in other chapters, consult with a health professional about how you can safely impact multiple conditions.

If you are taking medications—whether prescription or over-the-counter—or have any food restrictions, consult with your doctor before beginning any supplement program. Your health care provider should always be up-to-date on all vitamins, supplements, and herbal or homeopathic remedies you are taking. Supplement overdoses are rare, but possible, and certain combinations may affect individuals adversely.

Supplement	Dosage	Cautions
5-HTP	50–100 mg three times daily	Several months of treatment may be needed for maximum benefit. Nausea is the main side effect, but if it occurs, it usually dissipates within several days. Do not combine with prescription antidepressants. If you are taking prescription mediation for depression, you should consult with your doctor before taking 5-HTP. Excess levels of serotonin in the blood can be dangerous in case of coronary artery disease.
magnesium	Up to 1,000 mg	May take six weeks or more for effects to be felt.
melatonin	300 mcg–1 mg two to three nights per week	Tolerance may develop with regular use. Long-term effects of nightly use are unknown.

Supplement	Dosage	Cautions
vitamin B_2 (riboflavin)	Increase daily dosage from 50 mg to 150 mg. Do not exceed a daily supplement of 150 mg.	Must build up to a therapeutic level. May not show results for several months.
vitamin B_3	At the onset of migraine aura, take 100–150 mg.	High doses of niacin may cause a "hot flash" sensation. Some varieties are advertised as "flush free" and prevent this effect.

Alternative Health Remedies

When suffering from a specific condition like headache, we can also try some natural treatment options that are considered "alternatives" to traditional medicine. While a healthful lifestyle and the proper nutritional and supplement plan are vital to winning the battle against headaches, there are some other targeted remedies that might help, too.

Herbal Remedies

Some herbal extracts and homeopathic treatments have properties similar to conventional medications, but are gentler and may lack the drugs' side effects. Always inform your medical practitioner of any herbal remedies you may be taking.

- **Butterbur** is an herb native to Europe, Asia, and Africa. It is used in Germany to alleviate migraines. Butterbur's principal components are petasin and isopetasin, which are believed to slow the body's production of leukotrines—substances that can cause an inflammatory response and constricted blood cells. I recommend a daily supplement of 75 mg.
- **Feverfew** is an herb with anti-inflammatory and pain-relieving properties commonly used in Europe to impact migraine headache, especially the type with vomiting and sensitivity to noise and light. I recommend a daily dose of 250 mg.
- **Ginkgo biloba** enhances cerebral circulation and oxygen flow to the brain tissue. I recommend a daily dose of 120 mg, taken in two equal doses with meals. Ginkgo can act as an anticoagulant, and individuals

taking anticoagulant and antithrombotic drugs like ASA, anti-inflammatories, and warfarin or Coumadin should consult with their doctor before taking ginkgo.

- **Valerian** acts as a mild sedative and may play a role in helping to lower blood pressure. For migraine relief, I recommend taking 300–500 mg.
- **White willow bark** is commonly used in Germany as an alternative to aspirin for headache pain. I recommend taking 60–120 mg per day for relief of headache pain.

Homeopathic Remedies

The following remedies may be used for both temporary and acute cases of headache. When dealing with a chronic condition, homeopathic remedies must be used in conjunction with other therapies, as prescribed by a qualified health professional. Consult with your health care provider before taking any homeopathic remedy, and follow their recommendation for the appropriate dosage. Always inform your medical practitioner of any homeopathic remedies you may be taking.

- *Bryonia* is indicated when the headache is left-sided, over left eye or forehead, and worse when coughing.
- *Ferrum* is suggested for a continuous headache lasting two to three days. Headache can be in one spot on the left temple or a general frontal headache.
- *Gelsemium* is used for a headache that begins at the neck and gradually moves to the forehead.

Acupuncture

Acupuncture may provide relief from chronic headache pain. By listening to your symptoms and examining your appearance and pulse, acupuncturists can diagnose and impact headaches.

Acupuncture releases tension in the muscles. It causes a relaxation response in the body, resulting in lowered blood pressure and heart rate. Acupuncture increases the flow of blood, lymph, and nerve impulses to affected areas, and decreases stress while promoting feelings of well-being and energy.

Therapeutic Touch

There is a variety of treatments that involve the transfer of energy from the practitioner to the patient that can help to relieve pain and anxiety. In one study, massage reduced anxiety and lowered saliva cortisol levels (a key measurement of stress).[5] Massage can be very effective at removing tension from the muscles and may provide relief from headache pain.

REIKI Pronounced "ray-kee," this method employs a powerful hands-on healing technique in which the universal life-force energy is channeled through the practitioner and transferred to the patient. Chronic stress and anxiety can deplete the energy in our bodies. Reiki is used to support the body's natural ability to heal itself. It releases spiritual and emotional blocks, and brings a feeling of harmony and vitality.

MASSAGE This popular technique can enhance general relaxation and provide an outlet for stress and tension. Massage therapy can reduce feelings of anxiety, promote better sleep patterns, and increase feelings of well-being.

SHIATSU This form of physical therapy combines traditional Chinese medical theory and various Japanese massage techniques. The therapist uses direct pressure with hands and fingers to redirect the flow of energy throughout the body. Shiatsu treatment is deeply relaxing and can be beneficial in both chronic and acute conditions.

DENTAL DEVICES Many people who experience tension or migraine headaches also grind their teeth during sleep—a practice called bruxism. A device called an NTI-tension suppression system (NTI-tss) is created and fit by a dentist, and is worn while sleeping as a guard against tooth grinding and jaw clenching.

CRANIOSACRAL THERAPY This gentle form of manipulation is a hands-on healing technique that manipulates the craniosacral system— the soft tissues and bones of the head (cranium), the spine down to its tail (sacrum), and the pelvis, as well as the membranes and cerebrospinal fluid that surround these areas—to reestablish the normal flow of the cerebrospinal fluid. The practitioner uses an extremely light touch to palpate, or feel, areas to detect a fluctuation in the cerebrospinal fluid, and then manipulates the area to clear blockages and correct the flow. This therapy is beneficial in reducing stress, improving the quality of sleep, and enhancing the general functioning of the body's organs.

Neurofeedback

Also known as brain-wave training or EEG biofeedback, this technique is being used as a safe, drug-free alternative to impact stress, migraines, chronic pain, seizures, and more. Painless electronic sensors are placed on the scalp and earlobes. These sensors record the brain's activity, registering relaxed and focused brain waves with a video-game-like pattern on a computer screen. When the mind drifts, the screen goes blank. Neurofeedback is being used to reset particular brain patterns associated with certain illnesses or conditions, so the brain is able to perform at optimal levels. The effects that are experienced with the computerized biofeedback device are practiced and learned until the exercise and its effect on the brain can be reproduced at home without the device.

Aromatherapy

Essential oils can be used in baths or inhaled to provide rebalancing effects. Do not apply essential oils directly to the skin; they must be mixed with carrier oils. Some of the scents below may be effective in easing headache pain:

- eucalyptus
- ginger
- lavender
- peppermint
- rosemary
- sandalwood
- wintergreen

SUMMARY

The Mind Power program in this chapter stresses the importance of nutrition and lifestyle modification, both in preventing and impacting chronic headache. Remember, anything that impacts this disorder can be used to prevent it from occurring. Headache has many causes, and the appropriate treatment will vary from person to person. Addressing all aspects of physical, mental, and emotional health will help to prevent chronic and debilitating headache pain.

CHAPTER 10

BRAIN TRAUMA

Trauma to the brain can result from even the most mild of head injuries. In fact, approximately 80 percent of patients with traumatic brain injury (TBI) have the condition as a result of a seemingly innocuous accident or event.[1] Blows to the head, falls, automobile accidents, even whiplash can cause our brains to suffer harm sufficient to cause physical, mental, or emotional symptoms that range from moderate to severe.

Unlike some of the other conditions discussed in this book, there is not always something you can do to prevent an accident from happening. If you do have an accident that causes head injuries and possibly brain trauma, you must treat the situation with appropriate concern. Rehabilitation can be a long process, and your symptoms and needs may change as your recovery progresses. If you have suffered a trauma to your head, and are being treated for or recovering from a brain injury, you need to take it seriously. Consult with your doctor and be sure to inform them of any methods you are utilizing to speed recovery and support your brain's health.

In this chapter I will focus on ways you can help your brain to heal from a trauma, including which nutrients and supplements fortify and protect the brain, and alternative measures that may provide relief from some of the symptoms of brain trauma.

UNDERSTANDING BRAIN TRAUMA

Severe brain injuries can be permanently disabling, leaving the individual with a host of symptoms that must be addressed. More mild injuries, if left untreated, can also have serious consequences. Secondary cell death may cause wide and diffuse damage for months or years after the initial injury. The cortex, thalamus, and hippocampus, areas of the brain critical to memory and cognitive processing, are particularly vulnerable to such cellular decay.

In addition to ongoing damage to brain cells, one of the most serious aspects of TBIs is that the trauma not only kills or injures the brain cells—either at the time of the injury or during some interval thereafter—but also hampers brain plasticity, which is the ability of damaged brain cells to repair themselves.[2]

Studies have also established a link between TBI and Parkinson's disease.[3] Research shows that individuals who have suffered trauma to the brain may be more prone to Parkinson's disease. Individuals with TBI may also have a higher incidence of psychiatric conditions.[4] The study reported that the rate of psychiatric disorders one year after a TBI is considerably higher when measured against members of the general population who have not suffered a brain injury. Depression was found to be nearly seven times more likely in the brain injury group than in the general population.

Let's look at the areas of your brain that may be affected by trauma and the types of symptoms that may result.

Types of Brain Trauma

Trauma to the brain results in a variety of physical, mental, and emotional symptoms, depending on which part of the brain is injured. Following are some of the most common symptoms of brain trauma related to specific areas of injury in the brain.

Frontal Lobe (Forehead)

Trauma to the frontal lobe of the brain can result in difficulty with movement or paralysis. It can interfere with your ability to orchestrate complex or multiple movements. A person with injury to the frontal lobe may become fixed on a single thought, or be unable to concentrate while working on a particular task. They may have trouble finding the correct words or otherwise communicating with language. Emotional instability and personality changes are also characteristic of trauma to the frontal lobe.

Parietal Lobe (Top Back of Head)

An injury to the parietal lobe affects memory, causing sufferers to be unable to recall the correct names of objects or find the correct word when writing. They may experience difficulty in reading and simple mathematics. Difficulty in hand-eye coordination may occur, and drawing can be difficult. An individual with parietal lobe injury may be unable to discern left from right and often experiences extreme difficulty in multitasking.

Occipital Lobe (Back of Head)

Trauma to the occipital lobe commonly results in vision problems, including the inability to recognize colors, words, or the movement of an object. A person with an occipital lobe injury may hallucinate and may have trouble reading or writing.

Temporal Lobe (Above the Ears)

Injury to the temporal lobe of the brain causes short-term memory loss and may cause problems with long-term memory. Individuals may have difficulty recognizing faces and understanding spoken words. Fluctuations in an individual's sex drive may occur. Damage to the right temporal lobe may result in persistent talking.

Brain Stem (Deep Inside the Brain)

Injuries that cause trauma to the brain stem are very serious and often life-threatening. A decreased capacity for breathing may limit an individual's ability to speak. They may experience dizziness and nausea, problems with balance and movement, and difficulty perceiving and organizing their environment. Sleeping difficulties such as insomnia and sleep apnea may occur. More serious problems include the inability to swallow food or liquids.

Cerebellum (Base of the Skull)

Traumatic injury to the cerebellum causes the loss of fine motor abilities, tremors, dizziness, and even the ability to walk. It can cause an individual to have difficulty in reaching out and grabbing objects or making rapid movements. Slurred speech is a common symptom of trauma to the cerebellum.

Diagnosing Brain Trauma

Traumatic brain injury (TBI) happens when a sudden event harms the brain. Such trauma can be the result of an external blow to the head, such as might be suffered in a car accident, or when an object goes through the skull, damaging the brain tissue. When a TBI occurs and the skull has not been fractured, it is referred to as a closed head injury.

An accident does not have to fracture your skull or cause lacerations or broken bones, or even cause you to lose consciousness, for brain trauma to result. Whiplash or a seemingly innocuous blow to the head can cause serious injury, without you ever losing consciousness.

Traumatic brain injuries are usually rated as mild, moderate, or severe, depending on how long the symptoms last and whether you lose consciousness. But my contention is that any damage to the brain is serious damage and needs to be treated with appropriate concern. Hippocrates, the father of medicine, said it best: "No head injury is too severe to despair of, nor too trivial to ignore."

If you experience an injury to your head, a medical professional should carefully assess the level of trauma sustained by your brain. Experienced medical staff can stabilize your condition. In any head injury, it is crucial that the brain continues to receive the proper amount of oxygen and blood flow. This is important, both in treating the immediate condition of brain trauma and for your future brain health.

Being informed about the type of trauma to your brain will let you take preventive steps that will protect your brain as it heals and keep it healthy for a lifetime.

Symptoms of Brain Trauma

The symptoms of traumatic brain injury depend on the extent of the injury suffered. Such symptoms may include:

- persistent headache
- disorientation
- confusion
- light-headedness
- vertigo
- blurred vision
- ringing in the ears
- change in sleeping patterns
- mood or personality changes
- difficulty concentrating or maintaining attention
- memory lapses
- nausea
- seizures

- dilated pupils
- slurred speech

COMBATING BRAIN TRAUMA NATURALLY

Combating brain trauma naturally depends foremost on getting an accurate medical assessment of the type of injury the brain has sustained and the prognosis for the individual's recovery from a wide range of symptoms. A medical professional should immediately evaluate any head injury. A doctor can order X-rays, MRI, or PET scans and the tests necessary to determine the extent and seriousness of the injury, and can assure that the brain receives vital oxygen and nutrients immediately following a traumatic incident.

While you must follow your doctor's orders for treating a head or brain injury, there are certain things you can do to help protect your brain during this vulnerable time and speed healing and recovery. In the Mind Power protocol that follows, I recommend natural techniques for relief from symptoms of brain injury, as well as methods for revitalizing and rebuilding the vital brain connections that may have been interrupted by brain trauma.

Lifestyle

While no one can prevent every accident that may result in a traumatic brain injury, there are a few simple safety rules that can offer important protection against head injury:

- Wear helmets when participating in such sports as baseball, hockey, or horseback riding.
- Wear helmets when riding bicycles or motorcycles.
- Wear a seat belt when riding in a car.
- Make sure area rugs are nonslip to prevent falls.
- Use caution in the bathtub and shower; be sure to use a bathmat to help prevent falls.
- If you are experiencing dizziness or vertigo, consult with a medical professional to treat conditions that may cause a fall.
- Use caution when walking in slippery conditions like ice or snow or on wet floors. Older people can have difficulty with their balance and should be especially careful when the footing is treacherous.

Nutrition

What can be difficult in promoting proper nutrition as we age is the fact that our bodies may become less efficient in absorbing and utilizing key nutrients. Therefore, it is important that every bit of food you eat has the maximum positive impact on your mental health.

Foods and Brain Trauma

The proper nutrition can keep your brain strong and can help it to recover from damage from trauma. After a TBI, your brain is particularly vulnerable as it struggles to halt or repair cell damage. Diets rich in antioxidants can aid in the recovery of memory, halt brain cell loss, and improve the brain's function in all areas. Scientists believe the free radical cleansing effect of antioxidants is vital in preventing damage to the brain on a cellular level. In the nutritional plan provided in Chapter 2, I give you guidelines for a brain-healthy eating plan. To help your brain recover from an injury and help to support its return to optimal functioning, I recommend you review this chapter and the following plan for healthy eating, with a focus on antioxidant-rich foods.

Recipes

The recipes at the end of this book are intended to help you get started on a healthy eating plan that will provide optimum mental health benefits. Each dish focuses on foods rich in vitamins and nutrients beneficial to our brains. Eating right does not have to involve a huge effort. Prepare healthy dishes in larger quantities and store them for use throughout the week. In the list below are my recommendations for easy-to-prepare meals full of nutrients proven to help the brain recover from trauma.

Supplements

Even with a diet rich in recommended vitamins and minerals, your body may not efficiently absorb and process these necessary nutrients. As you grow older, your appetite may decrease, and you may find that you are unable to consistently take in the recommended amounts of food nutrients. It may be that getting these nutrients in supplement form is the most efficient way for you to enhance your healthy diet. However, supplements are not intended to replace healthy food choices.

Of course, before you begin any new health program, you should get a comprehensive, full-body evaluation performed by a qualified health care practitioner. A proper health and medical evaluation should evaluate your blood chemistry to assess your blood markers, your metabolic rate, and your blood pressure for indicators of cardiovascular, hormonal, or other imbalances or danger signs. If you are taking medications of any sort, for brain trauma or any other condition, you need to inform your doctor of any supplements you are considering adding to your daily diet, as some may interact with prescription medications and cause adverse effects. You should speak to your doctor before adding any of these supplements to your daily regimen.

Vitamins and Minerals

Certain vitamins and minerals are very important in protecting the brain from the symptoms of brain trauma.

LECITHIN/CHOLINE Choline, a key component of lecithin, is a building block of acetylcholine, a key neurotransmitter that may aid in brain-injury rehabilitation.[5] By encouraging brain wiring growth, acetylcholine can help the brain regain plasticity and repair damaged circuitry. Levels of acetylcholine are known to decline with age, and studies have shown that supplementation with choline can improve memory and learning. I recommend increasing your daily lecithin supplement from 1 gram to 2.5 grams for men and 2 grams for women. Take in two divided doses and do not exceed a daily supplement of 2.5 grams for men and 2 grams for women.

VITAMIN C In one study that examined the effects of free radical damage in patients with TBI, plasma levels of vitamin C were determined to be appreciably lower in patients with TBIs than in the control patients in the study. Furthermore, the vitamin C levels in TBI patients were inversely related to the diameter of the injury. In cases of brain trauma, I recommend increasing your daily supplement from 1 gram to 3 grams. Do not exceed a daily supplement of 3 grams.

Smart Drugs and Nutrients
Other naturally occurring nutrients may have beneficial impacts on the symptoms of brain trauma.

CURCUMIN According to a recent study, this antioxidant, found in foods like mustard and curry, has the potential to combat the effects of a TBI.[6] The study found that curcumin decreased the accumulation of damaging beta-amyloid proteins that can interfere with neural functioning in the brain.

Another study conducted at the UCLA labs looked at curcumin's protective benefits following a traumatic brain injury.[7] In this study, rats were placed on a curcumin-based diet for three weeks prior to experiencing a concussion, similar to that which an individual might experience in an auto accident. With this type of injury, most rats experienced a decrease in capacity for learning and memory. The brains of the rats maintained on the curcumin diet, however, were protected. To impact traumatic brain injury, I recommend a supplement of 500 mg taken three times daily.

NIMODIPINE Nimodipine dramatically improves blood flow in the brain by acting as a barrier to calcium in blood cells, allowing the cells to relax and raising the amount of blood and oxygen available to the brain. I recommend a daily supplement of 100 mg taken in four equal doses.

DMAE (DIMETHYLAMINOETHANOL) This nutrient, found in sardines, is a powerful stimulant that increases acetylcholine levels. Acetylcholine is an important neurotransmitter in the brain. It plays a role in memory, concentration, and focus. I recommend increasing your daily supplement from 150 mg to 650–1,650 mg. Do not exceed a daily supplement of 1,650 mg.

NAC (N-ACETYLCYSTEINE) This amino acid protects the brain from damaging free radicals by boosting quantities of glutathione, one of the body's most powerful antioxidants. I recommend a supplement of 500 mg taken three times a day.

PICAMILON Picamilon is used in Russia to treat brain inflammation, enhance cognitive abilities, and promote brain energy. Picamilon is a compound substance consisting of niacin and the neurotransmitter GABA. The niacin facilitates the passage of GABA through the blood-brain barrier, enhancing cerebral circulation and improving overall brain function. I recommend a supplement of 100 mg taken three times a day.

PS (PHOSPHATIDYLSERINE) PS helps the brain to use fuel more efficiently. It boosts neuronal metabolism and stimulates production of acetylcholine. As we grow older, aging slows the body's manufacturing of phosphatidylserine to levels that are detrimental to functioning at our full mental capacity. In the case of a brain trauma, it is even more critical for our brains to be able to access this vital neurotransmitter. To help your brain recover from a TBI, I recommend increasing your daily supplement from 300 mg to 400 mg. Do not exceed a daily supplement of 400 mg.

Mind Power Chart of Additional Supplements for Impacting Brain Trauma

The following chart summarizes the supplements I recommend adding to the protocol for overall brain health from Chapter 2. In some cases I recommend increasing the dose of a vitamin or supplement from Chapter 2 to impact a specific condition.

This protocol is designed for individuals who suffer from, or are specifically concerned about, brain trauma. If you are concerned about additional brain conditions discussed in other chapters, consult with a health professional about how you can safely impact multiple conditions.

If you are taking medications—whether prescription or over-the-counter—or have any food restrictions, consult with your doctor before beginning any supplement program. Your health care provider should always be up-to-date on all vitamins, supplements, and herbal or homeopathic remedies you are taking. Supplement overdoses are rare, but possible, and certain combinations may affect individuals adversely.

Supplement	Dosage	Cautions
lecithin/choline	Increase daily dosage from 1 gram to 2.5 grams for men and 2 grams for women. Take in two divided doses, and do not exceed a daily supplement of 2.5 grams for men and 2 grams for women.	Side effects may include nausea, bloating, vomiting, sweating, and diarrhea; extremely large doses can cause a heart-rhythm abnormality. Do not use if you have bipolar disorder.
curcumin	500 mg up to three times daily	
DMAE (dimethylaminoethanol)	Increase daily dosage from 150 mg to 650–1,650 mg. Do not exceed a daily supplement of 1,650 mg.	May be overstimulating for some people. Headaches, muscle tension, and irritability may occur. Do not take if you have epilepsy, a history of convulsions, or bipolar disorder. If you have kidney or liver disease, consult your doctor before taking this supplement.
NAC (N-acetylcysteine)	500 mg up to three times daily	Regular supplementation of NAC increases urinary output of copper. If supplementing with NAC for an extended period, add 2 mg of copper and 30 mg

Supplement	Dosage	Cautions
NAC (N-acetylcysteine) (*cont.*)		of zinc to your supplement routine.
nimodipine	100 mg taken in four equal doses	
picamilon	100 mg taken three times daily	If taking prescription drugs or MAO inhibitors, consult with your doctor before using.
PS (phosphatidylserine)	Increase daily dosage from 300 mg to 400 mg. Do not exceed a daily supplement of 400 mg.	
vitamin C	Increase daily dosage from 1 to 3 grams. Do not exceed a daily supplement of 3 grams.	

Alternative Health Remedies

When suffering from a specific condition like brain trauma, we can also try some natural treatment options that are considered "alternatives" to traditional medicine. While a healthful lifestyle and the proper nutritional and supplement plan are vital to winning the battle against brain trauma, there are some other targeted remedies that might help, too.

Herbal Remedies

Some herbal extracts and homeopathic treatments have properties similar to conventional medications, but are gentler and may lack the drugs' side effects. Always inform your medical practitioner of any herbal remedies you may be taking.

- **Ginkgo biloba** enhances cerebral circulation and oxygen flow to the brain tissue. I recommend a daily dose of 120 mg, taken in two equal doses with meals. Ginkgo can act as an anticoagulant, and individuals taking anticoagulant and antithrombotic drugs like ASA, anti-inflammatories, and warfarin or Coumadin should consult with their doctor before taking ginkgo.

Homeopathic Remedies

The following remedy may be used for both temporary and acute cases of brain trauma. Depending on the nature of the symptoms caused by a TBI, other homeopathic remedies may be appropriate to impact specific conditions, such as memory loss or depression. A qualified homeopathic practitioner will be able to advise you regarding specific remedies for impacting the aftereffects of a brain injury. When dealing with a chronic condition, homeopathic remedies must be used in conjunction with other therapies, as prescribed by a qualified health professional. Consult with your health care provider before taking any homeopathic remedy, and follow their recommendation for the appropriate dosage. Always inform your medical practitioner of any homeopathic remedies you may be taking.

- *Arnica* can help in controlling bleeding and swelling in the brain. It should be given as soon as possible after the brain injury occurs.

Therapeutic Touch

There is a variety of treatments that involve the transfer of energy from the practitioner to the patient that can help to relieve pain and anxiety, and may be helpful in promoting healing of a brain suffering from a traumatic injury.

REIKI Pronounced "ray-kee," this method employs a powerful hands-on healing technique in which the universal life-force energy is channeled through the practitioner and transferred to the patient. Chronic stress and anxiety can deplete the energy in our bodies. Reiki is used to support the body's natural ability to heal itself. It releases spiritual and emotional blocks, and brings a feeling of harmony and vitality.

SHIATSU This form of physical therapy combines traditional Chinese medical theory and various Japanese massage techniques. The therapist uses direct pressure with hands and fingers to redirect the flow of energy throughout the body. Shiatsu treatment is deeply relaxing and can be beneficial in both chronic and acute conditions.

CRANIOSACRAL THERAPY This gentle form of manipulation is a hands-on healing technique that manipulates the craniosacral system—the soft tissues and bones of the head (cranium), the spine down to its tail (sacrum), and the pelvis, as well as the membranes and cerebrospinal fluid that surround these areas—to reestablish the normal flow of the cerebrospinal fluid. The practitioner uses an extremely light touch to palpate, or feel, areas to detect a fluctuation in the cerebrospinal fluid, and then manipulates the area to clear blockages and correct the flow. This therapy is beneficial in reducing stress, improving the quality of sleep, and enhancing the general functioning of the body's organs.

Neurofeedback

Also known as brain-wave training or EEG biofeedback, this technique is being used as a safe, drug-free alternative to prevent stress, migraines, chronic pain, seizures, and more. Painless electronic sensors are placed on the scalp and earlobes. These sensors record the brain's activity, registering relaxed and focused brain waves with a video-game-like pattern on a computer screen. When the mind drifts, the screen goes blank. Neurofeedback is being used to reset particular brain patterns associated with certain illnesses or conditions, so the brain is able to perform at optimal levels. The effects that are experienced with the computerized biofeedback device are practiced and learned until the exercise and its effect on the brain can be reproduced at home without the device.

Prayer

For centuries people have been debating the efficacy of the role of prayer in healing. A scientific study, however, showed that those who prayed demonstrated healthier behaviors than those who did not.[8] Another study has shown that those in a test group who had a stronger belief in prayer had better physical functioning and higher mental health scores.[9] Traditional medicine may not point you in the direction of prayer: they prefer neatly boxed, quantifiable solutions to healing injuries. My feeling is that when an effective treatment for a condition is reported—whether it fits into the scientific box or not—it must be given some credit. When combating TBIs with alternative modalities, I urge you not to be afraid to think outside the box.

Hyperbaric Oxygen Therapy (HBOT)

Hyperbaric oxygen therapy improves the body's natural healing mechanism process by increasing oxygen levels in the blood. HBOT is a process of inhalation therapy that utilizes 100 percent oxygen in a total body chamber where atmospheric pressure can be increased and controlled. This direct delivery of oxygen allows the body's white blood cells to attack bacteria; it lessens swelling and enables new blood vessels to grow at a faster rate in injured parts of the body. HBOT can be used for both preventive and curative purposes.

Aromatherapy

Essential oils can be used in baths or inhaled to provide rebalancing effects. Do not apply essential oils directly to the skin; they must be mixed with carrier oils. Some of the scents below may be effective in easing the symptoms of brain trauma:

- chamomile
- geranium
- juniper
- lavender
- marjoram
- myrrh
- rose
- tea tree

SUMMARY

No two individuals will experience the effects of brain trauma in the same way. Treatment and rehabilitation will need to be tailored to specific symptoms and resulting conditions. If you have suffered a traumatic brain injury you need to support your brain's healing process with good nutrition and complement your doctor's prescribed programs and treatments with alternative healing modalities.

CHAPTER 11

BRAIN ALLERGIES

When I talk about brain allergies, I am talking about allergic reactions—most commonly triggered by ingestion of foods, food additives, or other chemicals—that affect the brain. Most people readily accept the assertion that what they eat can affect their bodies. What may be more difficult for them to believe is that food can have a strong impact on their brains. The fact is that our brains use approximately 30 percent of all the energy our bodies obtain from food.

Almost everyone has seen, or experienced firsthand, the effects of allergens. Dust, pollen, pet dander, and smoke are just some of the triggers that cause people to sniffle, sneeze, wipe at watery eyes, or break out in hives. As the scope of these symptoms show, allergic reactions can be manifested in any part of the body. Generally, allergies occur as a result of a hyperaggressive immune response that perceives a generally benign substance as harmful. The body tags the substance as harmful and white blood cells are mobilized to fight the perceived infection. In common allergic reactions, such as hay fever, a chemical reaction causes the release of histamines, which cause tissues in the eyes and nose to swell, causing the characteristic stuffy nose and watery eyes that accompany a hay fever attack.

What I want to specifically discuss in this chapter are allergic reactions that target the brain. These reactions are caused most often by particular foods or certain chemicals found in prepared foods. This type of allergic response is often difficult to diagnose, because the symptoms do not usually appear right after eating the offending food, but can take hours or days to manifest. The symptoms are not as easily diagnosed as the hives that might break out in a fixed allergic reaction to a single, particular food, like nuts, for instance. The symptoms of a masked, or cyclic, food-related brain allergy can be present as other brain conditions, such as depression, insomnia, mental fog, or even schizophrenia.

In the sections that follow I'll suggest ways in which you can identify and eliminate triggers for brain allergies, and tell you which nutrients and supplements will strengthen your body's immune system and your brain's capacity to resist an allergic attack.

UNDERSTANDING BRAIN ALLERGIES

When the response to a specific allergen has a detrimental effect on an individual's behavior, attitude, or emotions, it is likely that the sufferer is experiencing an allergic reaction in the brain.

There are certain biochemical reactions that are attributed to brain allergies, including excessive histamine release in the brain, alterations of levels of vitamins in the brain, changes in blood sugar levels, and neurochemical effects specific to certain food additives, such as NutraSweet, which contains phenylalanine.

Diagnosing Brain Allergies

The reactions to brain allergies can be extremely specific to each individual, with the same allergen producing very different symptoms in different people. But there are several methods for testing whether brain allergies are the underlying cause of certain medical or physical symptoms.

Brain allergies can be diagnosed using hair mineral testing, skin testing, blood tests that measure immunoglobulin food antibody levels and white blood cell reactions to antigens, and applied kinesiology. A method of removing specific foods or chemicals from your diet for a specific period of time before reintroducing them and noting the effect is a frequent diagnostic tool in testing for brain allergies. This "elimination diet" approach should be done under the supervision of a professional health care provider, especially if your symptoms are severe.

If you are undergoing a thorough medical workup to determine if you are suffering from brain allergies, I recommend you be tested for parasitic invasions, candida, and insufficient digestive enzymes. If any of these conditions exist, treatment can help improve your ability to absorb food nutrients and lessen systemic reactivity to certain foods.

Good dental care can play a role in reducing allergic reactions, too.

Infections hidden in root-canal-treated teeth, undetected abscesses, periodontal disease, or infection of dental implants can all trigger allergy-like symptoms.

Symptoms of Brain Allergies

Brain allergies can cause reactions that may present as diminished concentration, impaired thinking, spaciness, anxiety, headaches, aggressive or antisocial behavior, depression, rapid mood swings, insomnia, hallucinations, or episodic memory loss.

In children, brain allergies are thought to play a role in hyperactivity, learning disorders, and attention deficit disorders. In adults, manic-depressive disorders, hyperactivity, and various phobias may be symptoms of brain allergies. Severe psychotic reactions may occasionally occur. Food or chemical intolerances are thought to play a role in schizophrenia.

The effects of brain allergies are defined by both positive and negative reactions. An individual suffering from brain allergies might exhibit symptoms that vacillate between behaviors on both ends of the scale. This type of "roller coaster" of symptoms is a hallmark of brain allergies. In the scale that follows, the levels designated as positive (+) are levels of stimulation. The negative (−) levels are degenerative reactions.

- +4: mania, excitement, agitation, possibly convulsions
- +3: hypomania, anxiousness, aggressiveness, loquaciousness, apprehension, clumsiness
- +2: tension, thirst, talkativeness, argumentativeness, oversensitivity, hyperactivity, irritability, hunger
- +1: alert, active, lively, apparently symptom-free
- 0: homeostasis (even-keeled, in balance)
- −1: physical manifestation of runny nose, hives, gas, diarrhea, eye and ear symptoms
- −2: systemic reactions such as tiredness, mild depression, swelling, pain, cardiovascular effects
- −3: deepening depression, disturbed mental processes, confusion, moodiness, withdrawal
- −4: severe depression, possibly paranoia or suicidal tendencies

COMBATING BRAIN ALLERGIES NATURALLY

In individuals suffering from brain allergies, the delicate chemical balance of the brain has become hypersensitive to foods or environmental chemicals. Poor nutrition, stress, toxic metal poisoning, and environmental pollution may all serve to heighten the brain's sensitivity to allergenic substances. When treating brain allergies, all of these factors must be considered, in addition to removing the substance that is the primary trigger for the brain's allergic reaction.

Lifestyle

The best way to avoid allergic reactions is to stay away from the substances that provoke them. While I am specifically focusing on symptoms triggered by brain allergies in this chapter, if you are prone to allergic reactions in general, your immune system may benefit from specific allergen-removing techniques.

Removing Allergens from Your Home

Wash your bedding frequently in very hot water (at least 135°F) to remove allergens such as dust mites. Sheets, blankets, pillows, and comforters should be laundered weekly. Special covers that are dust-mite-proof and can easily be removed and washed can be purchased to go over mattresses and pillows.

Reduce allergens in your home and improve the air quality by using an air filtration system. Units with three to four filtering systems work best. These systems remove bacteria, mold, pollens, and animal dander from the air. Placing a filter directly in a window and sealing the sides will limit the amount of pollutants coming into a room.

Plants are also invaluable and inexpensive air filters. Spider plants will filter out toxins, including formaldehyde, and produce oxygen in return. Other helpful plants include Brazilian palms, wide-leaf wandering Jews, and marigolds.

New technologies such as ozone disinfection can purify water, including drinking water, saunas, whirlpools, swimming pools, and private bathing facilities.

Other steps you can take to remove allergens from your home include using natural, rather than chemical, products for daily grooming and cleaning:

- Use soaps without artificial scents or colors.
- Make homemade shampoos and conditioners using castile soap and olive or avocado oils; sesame oil makes an effective hair conditioner.
- Use peppermint and baking soda instead of commercial toothpaste.
- Use cornstarch instead of deodorant.
- Use cornstarch instead of talcum powder.
- Use sesame oil as a skin moisturizer.
- Use lemon oil and vinegar as room deodorizers.
- Use baking soda as a room or refrigerator freshener.
- Avoid the use of pesticides. Boric acid can be spread in a thin line (out of reach of children and pets) to discourage roaches and ants. In the garden, use insecticidal soap to kill pests without harming beneficial bugs.
- Create nontoxic surface cleaners using three tablespoons of vinegar to one quart of water for glass and smooth surfaces. Use baking powder instead of abrasive scrubs.
- In the laundry, pure baking soda will remove residues of detergent from clothing, and one cup of vinegar added to the rinse cycle will serve as a fabric softener and rinse out without leaving an odor. Look for natural detergents that do not have chlorine bleach or other chemical additives.
- Avoid dry-cleaning clothing whenever possible. If clothes must be dry-cleaned, remove them from the plastic cleaning bags and allow them to air out in the sun before wearing.

Nutrition

What can be difficult in promoting proper nutrition as we age is the fact that our bodies may become less efficient in absorbing and utilizing key nutrients. Therefore, it is important that every bit of food you eat has the maximum positive impact on your mental health.

Foods and Brain Allergies

If you suffer from brain allergies, you should avoid refined sugars and carbohydrates, caffeine and alcohol. Eat a diet with sufficient protein and make sure you get sufficient amounts of essential fatty acids from the right sources. EFAs have inflammation-fighting properties that are beneficial to allergy sufferers. Depending on what foods trigger your reaction, your diet must be carefully tailored to limit your exposure to certain foods. A clinical nutritionist can help you determine allergic triggers and create an eating plan that will reduce your allergic potential.

The most common brain allergy inducers are sugar, wheat, dairy, beef, potatoes, shellfish, eggs, tomatoes, coffee, peanuts, soy nuts, corn, yeast, and citrus. A rotation diet, in which different foods are eaten each day, without repeating any single item for four to seven days, can help you determine which foods may be triggers. If you have a slight sensitivity to a wide range of foods, this type of dietary approach can keep your body from overreacting to some foods. Others may have to be excluded from your diet on a permanent basis.

I recommend keeping a food diary in order to determine the specific chemicals and foods that produce allergic reactions. You should notice if you feel bloated or tired or if you have headaches after consuming particular foods. Even if these symptoms are not immediate, you should note them in your diary. If you are allergic to a food or additive, a pattern will begin to emerge.

Recipes

The recipes at the end of this book are intended to help you get started on a healthy eating plan that will provide optimum mental health benefits. Each dish focuses on foods rich in vitamins and nutrients beneficial to our brains. Because the reactions to foods that trigger brain allergies are so specific to each individual, there may be recipes below that are not right for you. If you find that you experience an allergic reaction after trying any of these recipes, eliminate that recipe from your diet until you can identify the ingredient causing the symptoms.

Eating right does not have to involve a huge effort. Prepare healthy dishes in larger quantities and store them for use throughout the week. In the list below are my recommendations for easy-to-prepare meals full of nutrients proven to help you prevent and impact brain allergies.

Head Cleaner, page 261
Relax Your Mind, page 263
Sleep Insurer, page 263
Fabulous Wild Rice Salad, page 266
Black Bean Soup, page 275
Chinese Mushroom Soup, page 276
Cinnamon Fruit Soup, page 277
Papaya Nectar Soup, page 279
Blueberry Breakfast Treat, page 279
Rice and Strawberries, page 281
Brazilian Rice, page 282
Good Shepherd's Pie, page 285
Blackberry Nectarine Fruit Salad, page 293

Supplements

Even with a diet rich in recommended vitamins and minerals, your body may not efficiently absorb and process these necessary nutrients. As you grow older, your appetite may decrease, and you may find that you are unable to consistently take in the recommended amounts of food nutrients. It may be that getting these nutrients in supplement form is the most efficient way for you to enhance your healthy diet. However, supplements are not intended to replace healthy food choices.

Of course, before you begin any new health program, you should get a comprehensive, full-body evaluation performed by a qualified health care practitioner. A proper health and medical evaluation should evaluate your blood chemistry to assess your blood markers, your metabolic rate, and your blood pressure for indicators of cardiovascular, hormonal, or other imbalances or danger signs. If you are taking medications of any sort, for brain allergies or any other condition, you need to inform your doctor of any supplements you are considering adding to your daily diet, as some may interact with prescription medications and cause adverse effects. You should speak to your doctor before adding any of these supplements to your daily regimen.

Vitamins and Minerals

CALCIUM To balance the effects of the magnesium supplement below, I recommend taking a daily supplement of 400–600 mg of elemental calcium from citrate.

MAGNESIUM Magnesium is well known for its calming properties in persons with anxiety symptoms, but proper amounts of magnesium are generally lacking in the average American diet. Individuals who use oral contraceptives or diuretics, who overuse laxatives, are at risk of magnesium deficiency. Magnesium also assists in impacting circulatory problems. For impacting the symptoms of brain allergies I recommend a daily supplement of 500 mg from citrate.

MANGANESE This essential trace mineral supports the immune system. Low levels of manganese may accentuate the symptoms of brain allergies. I recommend a daily supplement of 20 mg taken in two equal doses.

VITAMIN A Vitamin A is a great supporter of the immune system, and taking a daily supplement of vitamin A may reduce the possibility of developing allergies. I recommend supplementing with 10,000 IU daily.

VITAMIN C Vitamin C works to reduce histamine levels in the blood, detoxifies, and strengthens the immune system. I recommend increasing your daily supplement from 500–1,000 mg to 3,000 mg, taken in three equal doses. Do not exceed a daily supplement of 3,000 mg.

ZINC Zinc may fight food allergies by increasing production of hydrochloric acid in the stomach. Zinc also boosts the immune system. I recommend a daily supplement of 30 mg.

Smart Drugs and Nutrients

Other naturally occurring nutrients may have beneficial impacts on the symptoms of brain allergies.

BROMELAIN Derived from pineapple, this enzyme is a potent anti-inflammatory that helps to strengthen the immune system. To combat the symptoms of brain allergies, I recommend a daily supplement of 1,000 mg while the symptoms are present.

GLUTATHIONE A metabolite of the essential amino acid methionine, glutathione is an important part of the body's antioxidant defense system and enhances the immune system. To impact the symptoms of brain allergies, I recommend a daily supplement of 400 mg taken in two equal doses.

L-GLUTAMINE Glutamine is one of the most abundant nonessential amino acids in the bloodstream. It is produced in the muscles and is able to pass freely through the blood-brain barrier. Once in the brain, it is converted into glutamic acid and increases GABA, a neurotransmitter essential for proper mental function. There are two types of glutamine supplements: D-glutamine and L-glutamine. L-glutamine is the form that more closely mimics the glutamine in the body. For relief from symptoms of brain allergies, I recommend supplementing with 1,500 mg, taken daily in three divided doses while symptoms last.

METHIONINE Methionine is an essential amino acid and a powerful antioxidant, and helps protect the body from toxic substances as well as destructive free radicals. Methionine also acts to decrease the blood level of histamine, which, in brain allergies, can interfere with neurotransmitter messages. I recommend a daily supplement of 1,000 mg taken in two equal doses.

MSM (METHYLSULFONYLMETHANE) MSM contains bionutritional sulphur, which plays an important role in the body's functioning. It assists in restoring the immune system and also supports the respiratory system. I recommend a daily supplement of 1,000 mg taken up to three times daily.

Mind Power Chart of Additional Supplements for Impacting Brain Allergies

The following chart summarizes the supplements I recommend adding to the protocol for overall brain health from Chapter 2. In some cases I will recommend increasing the dose of a particular vitamin or supplement to specifically impact brain allergies. In these cases, you should increase the daily dosage from Chapter 2 to the level recommended for this specific condition.

This protocol is designed for individuals who suffer from, or are specifically concerned about, brain allergies. If you are concerned about additional brain conditions discussed in other chapters, consult with a health professional about how you can safely impact multiple conditions.

If you are taking medications—whether prescription or over-the-counter—or have any food restrictions, consult with your doctor before beginning any supplement program. Your health care provider should always be up-to-date on all vitamins, supplements, and herbal or homeopathic remedies you are taking. Supplement overdoses are rare, but possible, and certain combinations may affect individuals adversely.

Supplement	Dosage	Cautions
bromelain	1,000 mg daily while symptoms are present	
calcium	400–600 mg elemental calcium daily	
L-glutamine	1,500 mg daily in three divided doses while symptoms are present	Take while symptoms persist, but not for more than one month.
glutathione	400 mg daily in two equal doses	
magnesium	500 mg daily	May take six weeks or more for effects to be felt.
manganese	20 mg daily in two equal doses	
methionine	1,000 mg daily in two equal doses	
MSM (methyl-sulfonylmethane)	1,000 mg taken up to three times daily	
vitamin A	10,000 IU daily	
vitamin C	Increase daily dosage from 500–1,000 mg to 3,000 mg, taken in three equal doses. Do not exceed a daily supplement of 3,000 mg.	
zinc	30 mg daily	Large doses (50 mg or more) can interfere with the body's absorption of essential minerals, impair blood cell function, and depress the immune system.

Alternative Health Remedies

When suffering from a specific condition like brain allergies, we can also try some natural treatment options that are considered "alternatives" to traditional medicine. While a healthful lifestyle and the proper nutritional and supplement plan are vital to protecting the brain against allergens, there are some other targeted remedies that might help, too.

Herbal Remedies

Some herbal extracts and homeopathic treatments have properties similar to conventional medications, but are gentler and may lack the drugs' side effects. Always inform your medical practitioner of any herbal remedies you may be taking.

- **Astragalus** is one of the best immune system stimulants now available. I recommend taking 250 mg four times per day.
- **Chamomile** reduces inflammation by decreasing the body's production of histamines, prostaglandins, and other inflammatory agents. I recommend taking 325 mg three times per day, preferably with food.
- **Garlic** builds immunity and serves as a natural antiseptic agent. Add to your diet or take prepared capsules as directed by the manufacturer.
- **Goldenseal** was used by Native Americans for allergy or infection-induced conditions. Rich in alkaloids, it is stimulating to the immune system. I recommend taking 125 mg twice a day for three weeks at the first sign of symptoms. Note: Not to be used if pregnant or lactating.
- **Ginkgo biloba** is an extract of the ginkgo plant and is a potent antioxidant. I recommend a supplement of 120 mg per day taken in three equal doses.
- **Licorice root extract** has been used by the Chinese for over five thousand years to support the adrenal system. I recommend 100 mg taken one to three times daily. Note: Not to be taken if one has high blood pressure.
- **Marshmallow root** soothes inflamed tissues and contains key immune system boosters, including vitamins A and C. Marshmallow root is commonly taken as a tea, and should be prepared and ingested according to the manufacturer's directions.

- **Schisandra** is an adaptogenic herb that helps to rebalance the body, build strength, and reduce fatigue. I recommend 100 mg taken twice daily.

Homeopathic Remedies

The following remedies may be used for both temporary and acute cases of brain allergies. When dealing with a chronic condition, homeopathic remedies must be used in conjunction with other therapies, as prescribed by a qualified health professional. Consult with your health care provider before taking any homeopathic remedy, and follow their recommendation for the appropriate dosage. Always inform your medical practitioner of any homeopathic remedies you may be taking.

- *Conium maculatum* is useful in cases with impaired thinking, dull and sluggish mind, weakness of memory, and headaches.
- *Ignatia-homaccord* is a preparation containing ignatia and several active substances in a specific balance of potency.

Therapeutic Touch

There is a variety of treatments that involve the transfer of energy from the practitioner to the patient that can help to relieve pain and anxiety, and may be helpful in promoting healing of a brain suffering from an allergic reaction.

Craniosacral therapy is a hands-on healing technique that manipulates the craniosacral system—the soft tissues and bones of the head (cranium), the spine down to its tail (sacrum), and the pelvis, as well as the membranes and cerebrospinal fluid that surround these areas—to reestablish the normal flow of the cerebrospinal fluid. The practitioner uses an extremely light touch to palpate, or feel, areas to detect a fluctuation in the cerebrospinal fluid, and then manipulates the area to clear blockages and correct the flow. This therapy is beneficial in reducing stress, improving the quality of sleep, and enhancing the general functioning of the body's organs.

Detoxification

Many brain allergies can be traced to an impaired digestive system, which results from a toxic buildup in the intestines. An internal cleansing therapy can become the first step in overcoming the problems. The following detoxification programs should be undertaken only under the supervision of a medical health professional: bentonite clay detoxification; hydrotherapy, including colonic enema therapy; juice fasts (watermelon is a great detoxifier).

Aromatherapy

Essential oils can be used in baths or inhaled to provide rebalancing effects. Do not apply essential oils directly to the skin; they must be mixed with carrier oils. Experiment with some of the scents below to see if they bring you relief from symptoms of brain allergies.

- chamomile
- lavender
- lemon balm

SUMMARY

Over the years I have repeatedly emphasized the importance of the milieu—the environment of a person's body and immune system—in maintaining physical health on a cellular level. To protect your body against brain allergies and to combat the symptoms that may occur, it is important to protect your immune system by paying careful attention to triggers in your environment and foods. A strong immune system is your best defense against brain allergies.

CHAPTER 12

INSOMNIA

Sleep is an important part of our lives. While we sleep, our bodies are able to recharge and repair themselves at a cellular level. The effects of a lack of sleep are swift and apparent, especially as they relate to functions of our minds. Forgetfulness, irritability, lack of focus, and inability to concentrate are some of the most common manifestations of an exhausted brain.

It is not unusual to have trouble sleeping at times. But if you begin to consistently feel that you do not get enough sleep, or do not feel refreshed when you awaken, you may suffer from insomnia. Insomnia is the most common sleep complaint. Insomnia is not defined by the number of hours of sleep you are able to log per night. The amount of sleep needed to recharge each night varies from person to person; some people need less sleep, some need more, with the average "good night's sleep" being seven to nine hours per night. If you suffer from insomnia, you are not alone. Approximately 60 million Americans have trouble falling, or staying, asleep.

Insomnia is more common in women, especially those who have reached menopause, and in the elderly. You may have heard it said that as we age we require less sleep. Unfortunately this is not true. Our ability to sleep may decrease, but our bodies' need for rest does not. When you are dealing with insomnia, it is important to consider lifestyle, diet, and nutritional changes that will allow us to achieve the complete and restful sleep necessary for good health. In this chapter, I will offer some strategies for preventing and limiting insomnia, and show you how you can change your environment and diet to promote the type of sleep necessary for mental and physical health.

UNDERSTANDING INSOMNIA

Insomnia can encompass many sleep complaints, including difficulty falling asleep, difficulty falling back to sleep if awakened, sleeping too lightly, sleep disrupted by multiple spontaneous awakenings each night, or early-morning waking with an inability to fall back to sleep. Often insomnia is a symptom of an underlying physical or psychological condition. Let's look at the different types of insomnia and what causes them.

Types of Insomnia

Insomnia is categorized based on both cause and duration. It can occur as a result of one factor or a combination of factors that may be biological, physical, psychological, or environmental.

Primary and Secondary Insomnia

If a person is having sleep problems that are not directly linked to another health condition or problem, their insomnia is categorized as "primary." If they are experiencing sleep problems because of a physical condition (such as heartburn, asthma, arthritis, or restless leg syndrome), a mental condition (such as depression), or because of medication or other substances they are using (alcohol, caffeine), they are said to have "secondary" insomnia.

Transient Insomnia

Insomnia that lasts up to one week but then abates is called transient, or intermittent, insomnia. It is often caused by situational stress, such as that associated with a move, an upcoming deadline, or beginning a new job. People who suffer from transient insomnia often find it recurs with new or similar stressful situations. Good sleep habits and proven stress reducers are often effective in preventing transient insomnia, even when you are under stress.

Acute Insomnia

This type of short-term insomnia lasts for a week to several months and is usually associated with persistent stressful situations, like a death or serious illness of a loved one, or with environmental factors, such as noise, light, or extreme temperature. Acute insomnia may also be caused by changes in a normal sleeping schedule, like those experienced when switching from a day shift to a night shift at work, or suffering from jet lag.

Chronic Insomnia

Chronic insomnia occurs when a person has insomnia at least three nights a week for at least one month. It can be caused by many things, but most commonly occurs as a result of another health problem, such as depression, chronic stress, pain, and discomfort, such as that from arthritis. Heart disease, Parkinson's disease, sleep apnea, and hyperthyroidism are other serious health problems that may cause insomnia. Chronic insomnia can last for six months or longer.

Diagnosing Insomnia

If you think you have insomnia, you should talk to your health care provider. A medical history, physical examination, and sleep history will help to determine if there is a specific underlying cause. In the case of chronic insomnia, a psychiatric evaluation may be helpful in determining if your insomnia is a symptom of depression.

Keeping a sleep diary that keeps track of your sleep patterns and notes your perception of the quality and quantity of your sleep may be helpful in making a diagnosis. Be sure to provide your doctor with a list of all medications (both over-the-counter and prescription) that you may be taking. Some medications may contribute to insomnia.

Insomnia becomes more prevalent as we age, and most health care professionals look at four main areas when determining the cause of insomnia in older individuals:

- **Physical:** may include cardiovascular disease, asthma or other lung problems, chronic pain, bladder or prostate problems, epilepsy, sleep apnea, Alzheimer's disease or other dementia, and gastroesophageal reflux.
- **Environmental:** noise, late-night eating, late-night exercise, or inactivity during the day.
- **Medical:** drugs such as caffeine, alcohol, nicotine, antidepressant medications, stimulants, or medication schedules.
- **Mental:** depression (life changes and events that become more common as we age, such as retirement or death of a spouse or friends, may trigger depression), stress (health-related, financial), and anxiety.

Common tests to determine causes of insomnia may include:

- EEG sleep studies
- overnight oximetry (testing oxygen levels while you are asleep)
- mini–mental state exam
- cardiopulmonary exam
- neurological exam
- blood and urine tests

Symptoms of Insomnia

Insomnia is characterized by one or a combination of the following symptoms:

- difficulty falling asleep
- awaking often (more than three or four times) with a memory of being awake
- moving suddenly from sleep to wakefulness
- light, restless sleep that does not leave you refreshed, even if you sleep the same number of total hours as usual
- shifting sleep patterns (often a cycle of waking very early without being able to return to sleep, then having to go to bed earlier, causing even earlier morning wakings)
- confusion between day and night in terms of your body's levels of tiredness and energy

COMBATING INSOMNIA NATURALLY

Rather than becoming dependent on medications that induce sleep, it is important to prevent insomnia by making changes in your waking and sleeping habits and environment. For older people especially, the types of medications (called hypnotics) typically prescribed for insomnia can be metabolized at a slower rate, resulting in a rebound effect that may lead to carryover effects, such as daytime sleepiness, that could result in falls and injuries.

If your insomnia is caused by one of the underlying conditions addressed in the other chapters of this book, consult the relevant chapter for natural treatment options.

Quality sleep is essential in repairing and rejuvenating our brains and our bodies. In the Mind Power protocol for impacting insomnia that follows, I tell you how you can make your environment conducive to a restful night's sleep and suggest natural techniques for promoting relaxation and reducing stress. My nutritional and supplement plan in this section is specifically designed to prevent insomnia and allow you to get the optimal rest you need each night.

Lifestyle

There are three main areas that can impact our ability to get a good night's sleep. Our environment, our "sleep hygiene" habits, and our daytime activities are all factors in promoting or preventing insomnia. The suggestions below are proven insomnia fighters.

Environment

It is important that your nighttime environment is conducive to quality sleep. The following suggestions may help to prevent or overcome insomnia:

- Make sure your bedroom is dark, quiet, peaceful, and comfortable.
- Do not turn your bedroom into an office or den.
- Make sure your mattress is comfortable.
- Your bedroom should be well ventilated and slightly cool.
- Use a white noise machine or earplugs to cover any external sounds.

Sleep Hygiene

How you prepare for sleep will influence the quality of your rest.

- Avoid nicotine, caffeine, and alcohol late in the day.
- Avoid heavy meals late in the day. A light snack before bedtime may help regulate glucose during the night and help you sleep.
- Go to bed at the same time each night and wake up at the same time each morning. Avoid naps if possible.
- Do not go to bed until you feel tired.
- Follow a bedtime routine to help you relax before bed. A warm bath before bed can relax both your body and your mind.
- Avoid using your bed for any activities other than sleep or sex. Sex before bedtime may have the effect of either promoting or impeding sleep.

- Read or watch television (not in your bedroom, however!) until you feel drowsy. If you do not fall asleep after going to bed, get up again and engage in a nonstimulating activity (such as listening to relaxing music) for another half hour, then return to bed.

Daytime Activities

Your activities during the day can have an impact on the quality of your rest at night. To prevent insomnia:

- Exercise daily. Moderate exercise releases endorphins and natural cortisol, which reduce stress. Do not exercise in the three hours before your bedtime.
- Reduce stress by making a to-do list before you go to bed.
- Writing your worries in a journal can free you from worrying about them after you turn out the light.
- Practice relaxation techniques, such as meditation or breathing exercises, throughout the day so you are able to call on them at night when you want to "turn off" your stressful thoughts.

Nutrition

What can be difficult in promoting proper nutrition as we age is the fact that our bodies may become less efficient in absorbing and utilizing key nutrients. Therefore, it is important that every bit of food you eat has the maximum positive impact on your mental health.

Foods and Insomnia

If you suffer from insomnia, you should avoid any foods or beverages that may be stimulating, especially those that contain caffeine, sugar, or alcohol. To prevent any unnecessary stimulation to your system, you should avoid coffee, tea, cola, chocolate, spicy foods, refined carbohydrates, and prepared food with preservatives, especially those containing MSG. Sugar and foods high in sugar raise glucose levels and may create a burst of energy that disturbs sleep. Foods that are high in protein can inhibit sleep by blocking the synthesis of serotonin.

Do not combine too many ingredients in your last meal of the day, and avoid consuming too much food at night.

The best diet to promote a good night's sleep consists of a complex carbohydrate snack, such as whole grain breads, crackers, or bagels, which may help regulate glucose levels throughout the night, leading to a more restful sleep. Foods like turkey, bananas, figs, dates, yogurt, or milk are high in tryptophan—an essential amino acid that is a building block for serotonin—and may play a role in preventing insomnia. Niacin (vitamin B_3) is also involved in serotonin synthesis, and foods like barley, brown rice, tuna, salmon, cheese, and dried fruit are rich in this nutrient. Chlorophyll-rich foods such as leafy greens, chlorella, and spirulina may also help promote sleep.

Recipes

The recipes at the end of this book are intended to help you get started on a healthy eating plan that will provide optimum mental health benefits. Each dish focuses on foods rich in vitamins and nutrients beneficial to our brains. Eating right does not have to involve a huge effort. Prepare healthy dishes in larger quantities and store them for use throughout the week. In the list below are my recommendations for easy-to-prepare meals full of nutrients proven to help you prevent and impact insomnia.

Brain Juice, page 254
Chilling Relaxer, page 255
Chlorophyll Boost, page 255
Deep Sea Juicing, page 257
Free Radical Delight, page 259
Green Power Punch, page 260
How Green Is Your Juice, page 261
Relax Your Mind, page 263
Sleep Insurer, page 263
Fabulous Wild Rice Salad, page 266
Nature's Total Salad, page 272
Pasta Salad, page 273
Chinese Mushroom Soup, page 276
Blueberry Breakfast Treat, page 279
Cream of Barley, page 281
Rice and Strawberries, page 281
Brazilian Rice, page 282
Good Shepherd's Pie, page 285
Macaroni Marconi, page 287

Blackberry Nectarine Fruit Salad, page 293
Cherry Grape Kanten, page 295

Supplements

Even with a diet rich in recommended vitamins and minerals, your body may not efficiently absorb and process these necessary nutrients. As you grow older, your appetite may decrease, and you may find that you are unable to consistently take in the recommended amounts of food nutrients. It may be that getting these nutrients in supplement form is the most efficient way for you to enhance your healthy diet. However, supplements are not intended to replace healthy food choices.

Of course, before you begin any new health program, you should get a comprehensive, full-body evaluation performed by a qualified health care practitioner. A proper health and medical evaluation should evaluate your blood chemistry to assess your blood markers, your metabolic rate, and your blood pressure for indicators of cardiovascular, hormonal, or other imbalances or danger signs. If you are taking medications of any sort, for insomnia or any other condition, you need to inform your doctor of any supplements you are considering adding to your daily diet, as some may interact with prescription medications and cause adverse effects. You should speak to your doctor before adding any of these supplements to your daily regimen.

Vitamins and Minerals

CALCIUM Calcium can have a sedative effect on the body, and a calcium deficiency can cause restlessness and wakefulness. To impact insomnia, I recommend taking a daily supplement of 2,000 mg divided into four equal doses after meals and at bedtime.

IRON An iron deficiency may impact the quality of your sleep. If your doctor determines that you are deficient in this important mineral, I recommend adding a daily iron supplement of 15 mg for menstruating women and 10 mg for men and nonmenstruating women.

MAGNESIUM Magnesium is well known for its calming properties in persons with anxiety symptoms, but proper amounts of magnesium are generally lacking in the average American diet. Individuals who use oral contraceptives or diuretics, and who overuse laxatives, are at risk of magnesium deficiency. Magnesium also assists in impacting circulatory problems. If you are suffering from insomnia, I recommend a daily supplement of 1,000 mg taken in four equal doses, along with the calcium supplement.

Smart Drugs and Nutrients

Other naturally occurring nutrients may have beneficial impacts on insomnia.

L-TRYPTOPHAN A building block for the sleep-enhancing neurotransmitter serotonin, L-tryptophan may help to enhance relaxation and promote sleep. Tryptophan also enhances the brain's ability to produce melatonin, the hormone that regulates your body clock. I recommend taking 1,000 mg a half hour before you go to bed. If you awaken during the night and cannot go back to sleep, I recommend another 500 mg.

MELATONIN This hormone is produced by the pineal gland to aid in sleep and setting our circadian rhythms. Low levels can cause interrupted or restless sleep. To prevent insomnia, I recommend supplementing with 300 mcg–1 mg, taken a half hour before bed two or three nights per week.

Mind Power Chart of Additional Supplements for Impacting Insomnia

The following chart summarizes the supplements I recommend adding to the protocol for overall brain health from Chapter 2. In some cases I will recommend increasing the dose of a particular vitamin or supplement to specifically impact insomnia. In these cases, you should increase the daily dosage from Chapter 2 to the level recommended for this specific condition.

This protocol is designed for individuals who suffer from, or are specifically concerned about, insomnia. If you are concerned about additional brain conditions discussed in other chapters, consult with a health professional about how you can safely impact multiple conditions.

If you are taking medications—whether prescription or over-the-counter—or have any food restrictions, consult with your doctor before beginning any supplement program. Your health care provider should always be up-to-date on all vitamins, supplements, and herbal or homeopathic remedies you are taking. Supplement overdoses are rare, but possible, and certain combinations may affect individuals adversely.

Supplement	Dosage	Cautions
calcium (from citrate)	2,000 mg from citrate taken in four equal doses	
iron	15 mg daily for menstruating women; 10 mg daily for men and nonmenstruating women	
L-tryptophan	1,000 mg taken a half hour before bed. May take an additional 500 mg if awakened during the night.	
magnesium	1,000 mg taken in four equal doses along with calcium	May take up to six weeks for effects to be felt.
melatonin	300 mcg–1 mg taken a half hour before bed	Tolerance may develop with regular use. Long-term effects of nightly use are unknown.

Alternative Health Remedies

When suffering from a specific condition like insomnia, we can also try some natural treatment options that are considered "alternatives" to traditional medicine. While a healthful lifestyle and the proper nutritional and supplement plan are vital in preventing insomnia, there are some other targeted remedies that might help, too.

Herbal Remedies
Some herbal extracts and homeopathic treatments have properties similar to conventional medications, but are gentler and may lack the drugs' side effects. Always inform your medical practitioner of any herbal remedies you may be taking.

- **Chamomile** reduces restlessness and irritability at bedtime. I recommend taking up to 650 mg an hour before bed, preferably with a little food. Chamomile may also be used as a tea, taken in the hours before bed.

- **Skullcap** has a calming effect on the nerves and muscles and can act as a mild sedative. It may be particularly useful in easing the symptoms of "restless leg syndrome." Consult with your doctor if you are taking any other medications, including over-the-counter medications, such as antihistamines. If skullcap is safe for you to use, I recommend taking 1–2 grams up to three times daily. Skullcap is often combined with other mildly sedative herbs, including valerian, passionflower, hops, and lemon balm. If you are taking such a preparation, follow the manufacturer's instructions.
- **St. John's wort** is very popular in Europe, where double-blind, placebo-controlled studies support its efficacy in helping fight depression.[1] It has a calming and mildly sedative effect on the nervous system. To help impact insomnia, I recommend taking 450 mg twice a day.
- **Valerian** may help to improve sleep. It has a reputation for easing anxiety and relaxing tense muscles. I recommend taking 400–450 mg half an hour before bedtime. Do not take valerian for more than two consecutive weeks. Although the herb has no addictive properties, it is unwise to rely on any sleep aid exclusively. Valerian is often combined with other mildly sedative herbs, including skullcap, passionflower, hops, and lemon balm. If you are taking such a preparation, follow the manufacturer's instructions.

Homeopathic Remedies

The following remedies may be used for both temporary and acute cases of insomnia. When dealing with a chronic condition, homeopathic remedies must be used in conjunction with other therapies, as prescribed by a qualified health professional. Consult with your health care provider before taking any homeopathic remedy, and follow their recommendation for the appropriate dosage. Always inform your medical practitioner of any homeopathic remedies you may be taking.

- **Arnica** is good for insomnia brought about by physical overwork.
- **Aconite** is recommended in cases of insomnia caused by shock, grief, fright, or bad news.
- **Arsenicum Album** is for feelings of sleepiness during the day and restlessness at night.
- **Cocculus** is recommended when insomnia is brought about by overtiredness or exhaustion.

- **Ignatia** is used to prevent insomnia brought about by emotional stress.
- **Kali phos** is beneficial when insomnia is caused by excitement or mental strain.
- **Nux vomica** may be helpful when insomnia is caused by too much alcohol or food.
- **Pulsatilla** is recommended for early waking with an overactive mind and/or recurrent thoughts.
- **Sulphur** is suggested to treat night wakings followed by difficulty returning to sleep.

Acupuncture

Acupuncture may provide relief from insomnia. By listening to your symptoms and examining your appearance and pulse, acupuncturists can diagnose and impact insomnia.

Acupuncture releases tension in the muscles. It causes a relaxation response in the body, resulting in lowered blood pressure and heart rate. Acupuncture increases the flow of blood, lymph, and nerve impulses to affected areas, and decreases stress while promoting feelings of well-being and energy.

Therapeutic Touch

There is a variety of treatments that involve the transfer of energy from the practitioner to the patient that can help to relieve pain and anxiety. In one study, massage reduced anxiety and lowered saliva cortisol levels (a key measurement of stress).[2] Massage can be very effective at removing tension from the muscles and may provide relief from insomnia.

REIKI Pronounced "ray-kee," this method employs a powerful hands-on healing technique in which the universal life-force energy is channeled through the practitioner and transferred to the patient. Chronic stress and anxiety can deplete the energy in our bodies. Reiki is used to support the body's natural ability to heal itself. It releases spiritual and emotional blocks, and brings a feeling of harmony and vitality.

MASSAGE This popular technique can enhance general relaxation and provide an outlet for stress and tension. Massage therapy can reduce feelings of anxiety, promote better sleep patterns, and increase feelings of well-being.

SHIATSU This form of physical therapy combines traditional Chinese medical theory and various Japanese massage techniques. The therapist uses direct pressure with hands and fingers to redirect the flow of energy throughout the body. Shiatsu treatment is deeply relaxing and can be beneficial in both chronic and acute conditions.

CRANIOSACRAL THERAPY This gentle form of manipulation is a hands-on healing technique that manipulates the craniosacral system— the soft tissues and bones of the head (cranium), the spine down to its tail (sacrum), and the pelvis, as well as the membranes and cerebrospinal fluid that surround these areas—to reestablish the normal flow of the cerebrospinal fluid. The practitioner uses an extremely light touch to palpate, or feel, areas to detect a fluctuation in the cerebrospinal fluid, and then manipulates the area to clear blockages and correct the flow. This therapy is beneficial in reducing stress, improving the quality of sleep, and enhancing the general functioning of the body's organs.

Yoga and Meditation

Many have discovered the joy of yoga and meditation in helping clear the mind of thoughts and stress that can cause insomnia. Brief periods of meditation throughout the day can help refocus the mind and reinvigorate mental energy. The practice of walking meditation is particularly useful for achieving a restful state, as it combines both meditation and simple exercise.

To practice walking meditation, focus your attention on each foot as it contacts the ground. When the mind wanders away from your feet or legs, or the feeling of your body walking, refocus your attention. To deepen your concentration, don't look around, but keep your gaze forward and soft.

Aromatherapy

Essential oils can be used in baths or inhaled to provide rebalancing effects. Do not apply essential oils directly to the skin; they must be mixed with carrier oils. Experiment with some of the scents below to see if they bring you relief from insomnia.

- chamomile
- jasmine
- lavender
- lemon balm

- marjoram
- neroli
- rose
- sandalwood
- ylang–ylang

SUMMARY

In the sections above, I have focused on ways to impact insomnia when it occurs, but it is important to remember that insomnia itself is a symptom, not a disease. Insomnia is associated with a wide variety of mental and physical disorders, and these underlying conditions must be diagnosed and treated accordingly. Good sleep is crucial in supporting the functions and protecting the health of our minds and bodies.

CHAPTER 13

SENILE DEMENTIA

When people talk to me about growing older, they tell me that one of their greatest fears is that they will become forgetful. They fear that memory loss is the first sign of Alzheimer's disease and that it signals an inevitable mental and physical decline. For as long as I can remember—and for long before that—traditional medicine has told us that memory loss and confusion are simply normal parts of growing older. They implied that we should simply accept such changes in our mental capacities as an inevitable part of the aging process.

But I have known, and now modern medicine is beginning to admit, that remaining alert and able as we age can be the norm, rather than the exception. A lot of people experience memory lapses. Some are serious and others are not. People who have serious changes in their memory, personality, and behavior may suffer from dementia.

Dementia (from the Latin for "irrationality") describes a group of symptoms that are caused by changes in the way the brain functions. Senile (meaning old) dementia refers to the onset of these symptoms in older people. While dementia can strike anyone at any age, the most common conditions with dementia as a symptom include Alzheimer's disease and vascular disease, both of which are specific to older individuals.

By providing an optimal environment for brain health, and through a healthful lifestyle, attention to nutrition, and proper supplementation, you can preserve your mental abilities as you age. In this chapter I will talk about specific steps you can take to improve your environment and diet to protect your brain against the symptoms of cognitive decline associated with senile dementia. I will also talk about alternative, natural treatments that may have some benefits in the fight against this age-related condition.

UNDERSTANDING SENILE DEMENTIA

Individuals suffering from senile dementia have impaired memory as well as changes in other areas of cognition, such as language, vision, and abstract thinking, that prevent them from functioning properly on a daily basis.[1] The signs and symptoms of dementia occur primarily in the absence of delirium, and may be associated with an organic cause.

The classic indicators of dementia are short-term memory loss, inability to think through problems or to finish complex tasks, difficulty concentrating, confusion, and abnormal behavior.

While some types of dementia, such as that caused by Alzheimer's disease, often cause a steady and progressive decline in patients, other types of dementia can be prevented, treated, or reversed by addressing the underlying conditions.

Causes of Senile Dementia

There are many disorders that can cause dementia. Some, such as Alzheimer's disease, which accounts for approximately 60 percent of all dementia cases in the elderly, are characterized by steadily progressive loss of first cognitive, then physical, functions. Other causes of dementia are treatable and easily reversible, once the underlying condition is addressed. Reactions to medications, emotional stress, metabolic imbalances, problems in optical or auditory processing, nutritional deficiencies, hormone imbalances, diabetes, AIDS, Huntington's disease, head trauma, brain tumors, or inflammation or infection can all trigger symptoms of dementia. In the sections that follow, I discuss several of the most common conditions that can result in symptoms of dementia.

Alzheimer's Disease

This form of dementia encompasses a group of symptoms caused by changes in brain function. Alzheimer's disease is characterized by a specific, visible effect on the physical condition of the brain caused by the degeneration and death of neurons in the hippocampus. A sticky, waxy plaque called amyloid and neurofibrillary tangles are also present in the brains of Alzheimer's patients. For a detailed discussion of Alzheimer's disease, see Chapter 8.

Lewy Body Dementia

Lewy body dementia (LBD) is named after Frederick Lewy, who first discovered this form of dementia in 1914. LBD resembles Alzheimer's disease, but the abnormal brain cells, called cortical Lewy bodies, that are characteristic of this disease are found in the cortex and substantia nigra regions of the brain. Lewy body disease produces symptoms similar to Alzheimer's but may progress more rapidly.

Pick's Disease

Pick's disease affects the frontal and temporal lobes of the brain and is sometimes referred to as frontotemporal dementia (FTD). This illness is also similar in symptoms to Alzheimer's and generally affects individuals between ages forty and sixty. It is characterized by a gradual loss of social skills and personality alteration, as well as damage to the memory and language functions. Pick's disease is characterized in the brain by swollen neurons.

Vascular Disease

Vascular dementia is the second most common type of dementia after that caused by Alzheimer's disease. Vascular problems in the brain or body (most commonly strokes) are the main causes of this type of dementia. In general, this type of dementia occurs suddenly, frequently after a stroke. It generally does not progress steadily, however, like Alzheimer's-related dementia. The patient may have long periods of stability or even improvement, but quickly develop new symptoms if more strokes occur.

Pseudodementia

Some elderly people may suffer anxiety and fear that their mental abilities and memory are declining. These feelings may trigger a severe depression called pseudodementia. Cognitive changes, memory loss, and slowed motor movements are typical of this condition. This type of depression may also trigger other symptoms, like those of senile dementia, including apathy, inability to answer simple questions correctly, poor eye contact, or little spontaneous movement. Treatment of the underlying depression will cause the dementia-like symptoms to disappear.

Diagnosing Senile Dementia

Because there are so many conditions that have symptoms similar to those caused by senile dementia, and because there is no definitive test that can accurately diagnose dementia, diagnosis is often made by excluding other conditions that may present similar symptoms.

Symptoms of Senile Dementia

- forgetfulness at work
- difficulty with familiar activities; unwillingness to learn new things
- language problems
- problems with getting lost
- inability to keep track of days of the week
- impaired judgment
- problems with abstract thinking
- misplacing objects, or putting them in unusual places
- extreme or inappropriate mood swings
- personality changes
- paranoia
- loss of initiative, loss of interest in previously pleasurable activities
- motor skills impairment

Individuals suffering from the onset of senile dementia are usually unable to identify the problem themselves. If you or an elderly person close to you is exhibiting some of the symptoms above, a health care provider should be consulted and provide a thorough physical, neurological, and psychological workup as described in the following section.

A doctor will take a current medical and psychological history, assess neurological status, and evaluate physical status. You should tell your doctor about any medications or supplements you are taking. Some medications prescribed for other conditions can cause side effects that mimic dementia. Medical tests might include imaging scans, such as an MRI or CT; laboratory tests, such as blood and urine tests; neuropsychological tests, such as tests of memory, vision-motor coordination, and language function; and even a psychiatric evaluation to assess emotional factors.

It is important to remember that hormones are closely related to brain health. Hormone levels fluctuate with age, and the importance of consulting with an endocrinologist to assess hormone levels and balance in treating memory deterioration should not be underestimated. Hormones related to memory function include human growth hormone, vasopressin, DHEA, and pregnenolone.

To help your doctor rule out other causes of cognitive impairment, you should be prepared to discuss other possible causes of memory failure. Before settling on a diagnosis of senile dementia, carefully review the following areas with your doctor.[2]

- **Medication interactions.** Make a list of all substances you are taking, including prescription medications, vitamins, herbal supplements, over-the-counter products, such as aspirin or cold medications, smoking-cessation products, weight-loss products, and topical preparations, such as arthritis ointment.
- **Physical conditions.** Ask your doctor to ensure you are not dehydrated. Dehydration can occur from episodes of vomiting or diarrhea or from heat exhaustion. Dehydration is common in older adults, and can interfere with your body's ability to process medications or supplements.
- **Brain traumas.** Report any falls or blows to the head. Falls are common among older adults and can result in concussions and symptoms of dementia.
- **Emotional status.** The symptoms of depression can be remarkably similar to those of dementia. Discuss all possible triggers, such as loss, significant life changes, or side effects of medication, which may be underlying causes of depression.
- **Alcohol use.** Consuming too much alcohol or using alcohol with certain medications may cause memory loss.
- **Tobacco use.** Cigarette smoking is linked to changes in the flow of blood supply to the lungs and brain. Vascular disease is one of the primary causes of dementia.

COMBATING SENILE DEMENTIA NATURALLY

Remembering and forgetting things is a perfectly normal part of daily life. But we need not fear that the extreme and progressive cognitive decline that is a symptom of senile dementia will be an inevitable part of our aging process. There are a number of things we can do to positively impact our brain health and overall mental abilities as we age.

In the Mind Power protocol for impacting senile dementia that follows, I will tell you how you can make your environment more healthful, exercise your brain to retain memory and mental sharpness, and choose the best foods to help prevent the onset of senile dementia, or to slow the progression of cognitive decline if you have been diagnosed with this condition.

Lifestyle

Making healthful changes to your lifestyle can be crucial in preventing the onset of dementia and keeping your memory sharp as you grow older. There are several simple things you can do to prevent the onset of senile dementia or to slow or prevent the progression of symptoms. In the sections below, I offer suggestions for improving your living environment, your physical health, and your social support system—changes that can help you fight age-related memory loss and dementia. I have even included some coping strategies to make short-term memory loss less disruptive in your daily routine.

Environment

It is important for your environment to be free of hazardous toxins, particularly heavy metals, that can accumulate in the body. Limit your exposure to cookware, deodorants, antacids, and food additives that contain aluminum. Mercury is found in thermometers, thermostats, and dental amalgams. Chelation therapy, which uses certain amino acids to form strong ionic bonds with the toxic metals in your body, allowing them to be excreted from the system, may be useful in removing toxic metals and other chemicals from your body. (If you are interested in finding out more about chelation therapy, read the article posted on my Web site at www.garynull.com/ Documents/Chelation_Therapy.htm.) Bentonite, a claylike substance that is used in a drink, may be taken at night to draw out toxins from the colon and assist in the detoxification process.

Installing charcoal filters on all water sources used for drinking or cooking can reduce or eliminate harmful toxins that are found in the water from our reservoirs.

Social Activity

Continued community involvement and frequent contact with friends and family may reduce your risk for senile dementia. In a paper presented at the Alzheimer's Association International Conference on the Prevention of Dementia,[3] Jane Saczynski, Ph.D., of the National Institute on Aging, and colleagues presented data from a longitudinal study, conducted since 1965, that showed that subjects with decreased social activity from mid- to late life had a statistically significant risk of dementia. Continue to set goals for yourself. Having a reason to get up and get going each day can enhance your overall quality of life and contribute to mental fitness.

Exercise

Physical activity seems to play a role in slowing or preventing the progression of senile dementia. A National Institutes of Health news release cites research demonstrating that long-term physical activity increased the learning ability of mice and decreased the level of plaque-forming beta-amyloid protein fragments in their brains.[4] Remaining physically active throughout our lifetimes offers immeasurable benefits to both body and brain. Physical activity does not have to be rigorous. Walking, dancing, or practicing yoga all help safeguard our brains against age-related cognitive decline.

Memory Skills and Brain Boosters

In addition to an active body, it is important to have an active mind. A study published in the *New England Journal of Medicine* supports the theory that mentally demanding activities can help stave off dementia.[5] The study involved 469 people aged seventy-five and older. Those participants who read, played games of strategy, such as checkers, backgammon, or chess, played musical instruments, or danced at least twice a week were significantly less likely to develop dementia. Those who did crossword puzzles four times a week were also found to have a significantly lowered risk. It seems clear that participating in mentally stimulating hobbies and being willing to learn new information and challenge our brains on an ongoing basis provide important benefits in preventing the onset of senile dementia.

Weight Management

A recent study published in the *British Medical Journal* examined more than 10,000 members of a medical insurance program in California. The study followed subjects from their early forties until their late sixties and seventies. According to the results, those individuals who were obese at the start of the study were 74 percent more likely to develop dementia than their slimmer counterparts.[6]

Coping Strategies

If you or someone close to you has been diagnosed as having senile dementia, there are some strategies for coping with the symptoms of memory loss that may be the first hallmarks of this disease. These coping strategies will help relieve the stress and tension that arise from memory problems, and can help lessen the impact of such problems on day-to-day life. Remember, in addition to practicing the strategies outlined below, you should make the lifestyle and nutritional changes I recommend in this chapter to slow or reverse the progression of these early symptoms.

- Establish a regular routine in familiar surroundings.
- Make mental associations, such as using landmarks, to help you find things.
- Repeat names when you meet people.
- Put important items, such as your keys, in the same place every time.
- Label or color-code doors and exits to keep from getting disoriented.
- Draw a map for simple routes; write down directions.
- Make lists, use a calendar, and keep notes of important dates and financial matters.
- Set realistic daily goals.
- Keep track of when medicines are taken; use a chart or special pill box to stay current.
- Tell your doctor about all medications or supplements you are taking.
- Keep a list of important names and numbers near the telephone.
- Stay in frequent contact with family and friends.

Nutrition

What can be difficult in promoting proper nutrition as we age is the fact that our bodies may become less efficient in absorbing and utilizing key nutrients. Therefore, it is important that every bit of food you eat has the maximum positive impact on your mental health.

Foods and Senile Dementia

As research into the causes of dementia continues, researchers are concluding that there may be ways in which we can limit our risk of developing senile dementia as we age. What is now being proposed is something that I have said over and over again: deficiencies of essential nutrients can lead to a variety of health problems and leave us vulnerable to serious conditions such as senile dementia. The good news is that it is never too early to start good nutritional habits that will help to protect the brain over a lifetime. And it is never too late to benefit from good nutritional habits.

Most Americans today eat foods that are overprocessed and far from their natural state. These processed foods have been stripped of vital nutrients and filled with additives, processed sugars, and trans fats.

In addition to nutrients lost through poor diet, nutritional deficiencies may simply increase as we age. To help ensure that our bodies get the nutrients we need, we must make an effort to eat foods in their natural state. For people suffering from senile dementia it is vitally important to purchase organic foods whenever possible, since these foods are more likely to have trace minerals like chromium, magnesium, selenium, and zinc, which are vital to the brain's health.

Various studies support the efficacy of taking antioxidants as a method of preventing or reversing cognitive decline. Vitamins E and C are proven free radical fighters and readily available in foods like citrus fruits and juices, dark green, leafy vegetables, nuts, and sunflower seeds. The B vitamins, which play an important role in fighting the symptoms of Alzheimer's disease, are found in fish, eggs, beans, and animal proteins. Trace minerals like zinc, magnesium, and potassium are easy to add to our diets by using whole grains, nuts, dried beans, bananas, and milk.

Essential fatty acids (EFAs) such as omega-3 and omega-6 fats, which are found in cold-water fish like salmon, mackerel, sardines, and herring, as well as in flax oil, walnuts, and oysters, have significant anti-inflammatory properties and may be important in preventing senile dementia.

Recipes

The recipes at the end of this book are intended to help you get started on a healthy eating plan that will provide optimum mental health benefits. Each dish focuses on foods rich in vitamins and nutrients beneficial to our brains. Eating right does not have to involve a huge effort. Prepare healthy dishes in larger quantities and store them for use throughout the week. In the list below are my recommendations for easy-to-prepare meals full of nutrients proven to help prevent the onset of senile dementia.

Antioxidant Punch, page 252
Blueberry and Pear Macadamia Nut Shake, page 253
Brain Power, page 254
Carrot, Pineapple, and Strawberry Juice, page 254
Everglades Punch, page 258
Flax Cruncher, page 259
Free Radical Delight, page 259
Nuts and Seeds, page 262
Velvety Pecan Milk, page 265
Four Bean Salad, page 266
Mixed Sprout, Bean, and Nut Salad, page 271
Black Bean Soup, page 275
Cream of Barley, page 281
Nutty Oatmeal, page 281
Gary's Veggieball Stew, page 284
Indonesian Kale, page 286
Pasta Fagioli, page 288
Sweet Kidney Bean Mash, page 290
Heavenly Roasted Nuts, page 296

Supplements

Even with a diet rich in recommended vitamins and minerals, your body may not efficiently absorb and process these necessary nutrients. As you grow older, your appetite may decrease, and you may find that you are unable to consistently take in the recommended amounts of food nutrients. It may be that getting these nutrients in supplement form is the most efficient way for you to enhance your healthy diet. However, supplements are not intended to replace healthy food choices.

Of course, before you begin any new health program, you should get a comprehensive, full-body evaluation performed by a qualified health care practitioner. A proper health and medical evaluation should evaluate your blood chemistry to assess your blood markers, your metabolic rate, and your blood pressure for indicators of cardiovascular, hormonal, or other imbalances or danger signs. If you are taking medications of any sort, for senile dementia or any other condition, you need to inform your doctor of any supplements you are considering adding to your daily diet, as some may interact with prescription medications and cause adverse effects. You should speak to your doctor before adding any of these supplements to your daily regimen.

Vitamins and Minerals

Certain vitamins and minerals are very important in fighting the onset of senile dementia.

CALCIUM Calcium from citrate can have a calming effect on the body, and a calcium deficiency can cause restlessness and wakefulness. To impact restlessness associated with senile dementia, I recommend taking a daily supplement of 1,000 mg divided into four equal doses after meals and at bedtime.

MAGNESIUM Magnesium is well known for its calming properties in persons with anxiety symptoms, but proper amounts of magnesium are generally lacking in the average American diet. Individuals who use oral contraceptives or diuretics, and who overuse laxatives, are at risk of magnesium deficiency. Magnesium from citrate also assists in impacting circulatory problems. I recommend a daily supplement of 500–1,000 mg of magnesium taken in two equal doses on an empty stomach.

POTASSIUM Potassium is one of the most abundant minerals in the human body. Most of the time supplementation with potassium is unnecessary, because it is so readily available in our diet in such foods as bananas, orange juice, and potatoes. Potassium is depleted from our bodies in times of stress, thus upsetting the delicate balance of neurotransmitter communication in our brains. For this reason, potassium supplements may be useful in impacting senile dementia. Potassium can interact with some drugs, so if you are taking prescription medications, consult with your doctor before taking potassium supplements. If potassium is safe for you, I recommend a daily supplement of 500 mg.

VITAMIN B COMPLEX It is important that your daily vitamin B complex contain sufficient amounts of both vitamin B_5 and B_{12}, as deficiencies in these vitamins can develop as we age, and these deficiencies can contribute to the symptoms of senile dementia. If your doctor has determined you are deficient in B vitamins, you may want to ask about receiving intravenous or injected supplements of vitamin B complex to prevent or combat symptoms of senile dementia.

VITAMIN C Vitamin C may help delay the onset of senile dementia and slow the progression of symptoms. I recommend increasing your daily supplement from 500–1,000 mg to 3,000 mg, taken in three equal doses. Do not exceed a daily supplement of 3,000 mg.

VITAMIN E Vitamin E has beneficial antioxidant properties, and treatment with high doses has shown initial promise in slowing the progression of symptoms in individuals with dementia associated with moderately severe Alzheimer's.[7] Because vitamin E has anticoagulant properties, and high doses may be associated with the risk of bleeding and interaction with anticoagulants and other medications often taken by elderly people, you should discuss high-dose vitamin E supplementation with your doctor. If you are not at risk, I recommend increasing your daily supplement from 400 IU to 800 IU, taken in two equal doses. Do not exceed a daily supplement of 800 IU.

ZINC Many people who suffer from dementia have deficiencies in zinc. I recommend a daily supplement of 30 mg.

Smart Drugs and Nutrients

A number of other naturally occurring nutrients may have beneficial impacts on the symptoms of senile dementia.

ACETYL-L-CARNITINE (ACL) This versatile nutrient is able to permeate the blood-brain barrier to stimulate and fortify the brain's nerve cells. Acetyl-L-carnitine is a type of carnitine produced naturally in the brain. It can aid in directing fatty acids to the cell mitochondria, assisting in the creation of new cell energy. A powerful antioxidant, acetyl-L-carnitine also supplements the neurotransmitter acetylcholine. I recommend increasing your daily supplement from 2,000 mg to 3,000 mg, taken in three equal doses. Do not exceed a daily supplement of 3,000 mg.

L-GLUTAMINE Glutamine is one of the most abundant nonessential amino acids in the bloodstream. It is produced in the muscles and is able to pass freely through the blood-brain barrier. Once in the brain, it is converted into glutamic acid and increases GABA, a neurotransmitter essential for proper mental function. There are two types of glutamine supplements: D-glutamine and L-glutamine. L-glutamine is the form that more closely mimics the glutamine in the body. To impact the symptoms of senile dementia, I recommend supplementing with 500 mg taken three times daily.

NAC (N-ACETYLCYSTEINE) This amino acid protects the brain from damaging free radicals by boosting quantities of glutathione, one of the body's most powerful antioxidants. I recommend a supplement of 500 mg taken three times daily.

PS (PHOSPHATIDYLSERINE) PS helps the brain use fuel more efficiently. By boosting neuronal metabolism and stimulating production of acetylcholine, PS may be able to improve the condition of patients in cognitive decline. Studies have revealed that supplementing with phosphatidylserine slows down—and even reverses—declining memory and concentration, or age-related cognitive impairment in middle-aged and elderly subjects.[8]

As we grow older, aging slows the body's manufacturing of phosphatidylserine to levels that are detrimental to our functioning at our full mental capacity. For treatment of memory loss that accompanies senile dementia, I recommend increasing your daily supplement from 300 mg to 400 mg. Do not exceed a daily supplement of 400 mg.

SAME (S-ADENOSYLMETHIONINE) SAMe (pronounced "sammy") has long been prescribed by European doctors as a treatment for depression. SAMe promotes cell growth and repair, and maintains levels of glutathione, a major antioxidant that protects against free radicals and reduces homocysteine levels. Alzheimer patients have extremely low levels of SAMe in their brains. SAMe should not be taken if you are taking MAO inhibitor antidepressants. You should consult with your doctor before taking SAMe if you suffer from severe depression or bipolar disorder. If SAMe is safe for you to use, I recommend a daily supplement of 400–1,600 mg, taken in four equal doses.

Mind Power Chart of Additional Supplements for Impacting Senile Dementia

The following chart summarizes the supplements I recommend adding to the protocol for overall brain health from Chapter 2. In some cases I will recommend increasing the dose of a particular vitamin or supplement to specifically impact senile dementia. In these cases, you should increase the daily dosage from Chapter 2 to the level recommended for this specific condition.

This protocol is designed for individuals who suffer from, or are specifically concerned about, senile dementia. If you are concerned about additional brain conditions discussed in other chapters, consult with a health professional about how you can safely impact multiple conditions.

If you are taking medications—whether prescription or over-the-counter—or have any food restrictions, consult with your doctor before beginning any supplement program. Your health care provider should always be up-to-date on all vitamins, supplements, and herbal or homeopathic remedies you are taking. Supplement overdoses are rare, but possible, and certain combinations may affect individuals adversely.

Supplement	Dosage	Cautions
acetyl-L-carnitine (ACL)	Increase daily dosage from 2,000 mg to 3,000 mg, taken in three equal doses. Do not exceed a daily supplement of 3,000 mg.	
calcium	1,000 mg daily in four equal doses after meals and at bedtime	
intravenous vitamin B complex	Discuss with your health care provider whether you might benefit from injected vitamin B.	
L-glutamine	500 mg taken three times daily	
magnesium	500–1,000 mg in two equal doses	May take up to six weeks for effects to be felt. Take on an

continued...

Supplement	Dosage	Cautions
magnesium (*cont.*)		empty stomach. If loose stools occur, decrease dosage.
NAC (N-acetylcysteine)	500 mg three times daily	Regular supplementation of NAC increases urinary output of copper. If supplementing with NAC for an extended period, add 2 mg of copper and 30 mg of zinc to your daily supplement regimen.
PS (phosphatidylserine)	Increase daily dosage from 300 mg to 400 mg. Do not exceed a daily supplement of 400 mg.	
potassium	500 mg daily	Do not take potassium supplements if you are taking medication for high blood pressure or heart disease, or if you have a kidney disorder. Consuming foods rich in potassium is okay. Do not exceed a supplementary dose of 500 mg daily without consulting your doctor.
SAMe (S-adenosylmethionine)	dosage range of 400–1,600 mg	Raise the dose gradually from 200 mg twice a day to 400 mg twice a day, to 400 mg three times a day, to 400 mg four times a day, over a period of twenty days.
vitamin C	Increase daily dosage from 500–1,000 mg to 3,000 mg, taken in three equal doses. Do not exceed a daily supplement of 3,000 mg.	

Supplement	Dosage	Cautions
vitamin E	Increase daily dosage from 400 IU to 800 IU, taken in two equal doses. Do not exceed a daily supplement of 800 IU.	Vitamin E may cause increased risk of bleeding and may have adverse interactions with anticoagulants or other medications. Consult with your doctor before beginning high-dose supplementation with vitamin E.
zinc	Up to 30 mg daily	Large doses (50 mg or more) can interfere with the body's absorption of essential minerals, impair blood cell function, and depress the immune system.

Alternative Health Remedies

When suffering from a condition like senile dementia, we can also try some natural treatment options that are considered "alternatives" to traditional medicine. While a healthful lifestyle and the proper nutritional and supplement plan are vital to winning the battle against dementia, there are some other targeted remedies that might help, too.

Herbal Remedies

Some herbal extracts and homeopathic treatments have properties similar to conventional medications, but are gentler and may lack the drugs' side effects. Always inform your medical practitioner of any herbal remedies you may be taking.

- **Butcher's broom** is an herb that promotes clearer focus and enhanced memory. I recommend a daily supplement of 850 mg taken in two equal doses.
- *Bacopa monnieri* is a potent antioxidant that has been used in Ayurvedic medicine for centuries as a brain tonic to enhance memory, learning, development, and concentration. I recommend a daily supplement of 200–400 mg taken in two equal doses.

- **Ginkgo biloba** is an herbal extract derived from the ginkgo biloba tree. It is commonly used in Europe to combat Alzheimer's disease. Ginkgo biloba is a potent antioxidant that may be beneficial in impacting dementia-related symptoms. By improving circulation to the central nervous system, ginkgo biloba may help to stabilize abnormal neurotransmitter communication in the brain. In a study conducted at the New York Institute for Medical Research, researchers found that almost one-third of Alzheimer's patients taking ginkgo supplements showed improvements in cognitive function during a double-blind, placebo-controlled clinical study.[9] For prevention of senile dementia, I recommend a daily supplement of 120 mg taken in two equal doses. For those suffering from this condition, I recommend increasing your daily dose to 240 mg, spread out over three equal doses.

- **KUT** (*Kami-Untan-To*) is a Japanese herbal medicine that has been used for centuries in Japan to help with neuropsychiatric problems. In animal studies KUT has been shown to increase choline acetyltransferase levels and nerve growth factor.[10] Later studies showed that KUT may be beneficial as an interventional strategy to fight senile dementia by slowing cognitive decline.[11] KUT is a combination of thirteen different herbs and should be taken as directed by the manufacturer.

- **Huperzine A** is a compound isolated from a Chinese herb called *Hyperzia serrata*. It increases acetylcholine activity in the cortex and hippocampus sections of the brain, and aids in improving memory as well as cognitive and behavioral functions. In a double-blind, placebo-controlled study conducted in China, 103 individuals with Alzheimer's disease received either huperzine A or a placebo twice daily for eight weeks. About 60 percent of the participants treated with huperzine A showed significant improvements in memory, thinking, and behavioral functions, compared to 36 percent of the placebo-treated subjects.[12] For impacting senile dementia, I recommend taking a daily supplement of 100–200 mcg in two equal doses.

- **St. John's wort** (*Hypericum*) is very popular in Europe, so much so that it is actually covered by German health insurance as a prescription drug. I recommend taking a daily supplement of 300 mg twice per day.

- **Vinpocetine** is a derivative of an extract taken from the periwinkle shrub. It enhances circulation to the brain, and may prevent or improve mild cognitive impairment. I recommend taking 10 mg twice daily with meals.

Homeopathic Remedies

The following remedies may be used for both temporary and acute cases of senile dementia. When dealing with a chronic condition, homeopathic remedies must be used in conjunction with other therapies, as prescribed by a qualified health professional. Consult with your health care provider before taking any homeopathic remedy, and follow their recommendation for the appropriate dosage. Always inform your medical practitioner of any homeopathic remedies you may be taking.

- *Alumina* is indicated for impacting great weakness or loss of memory in cases where consciousness of personal identity is confused.
- *Anacardium* is used for absentmindedness; memory for names is most affected.
- *Argentum nitricum* is for dementia with irritability and lack of control over impulses.
- *Helleborus* impacts stupefaction, when a person answers questions slowly and stares vacantly.
- *Silica* is best for mental deterioration with anxiety over small details.
- **Sulphur** can be used when there is difficulty remembering words or names.

Aromatherapy

Essential oils can be used in baths or inhaled to provide an energizing or soothing effect. Do not apply essential oils directly to the skin; they must be mixed with carrier oils. Experiment with various scents to see which help to alleviate the symptoms of senile dementia and increase mental clarity.

- bergamot
- clove
- frankincense
- lavender
- lemon balm

SUMMARY

Contrary to mainstream medical belief, there are safe, natural, and nontoxic treatments that can alleviate the symptoms of senile dementia. Research has demonstrated how these remedies can aid in preventing the onset of senile dementia. In the past, dementia was considered an uncontrollable outcome of aging. Taking action now can prevent our elder years from being characterized by cognitive degeneration and a rapid decline in health and ability.

CHAPTER 14

PSYCHONEUROIMMUNOLOGY

The greatest discovery of my generation is that man can alter his life simply by altering his attitude of mind.

—William James

Man is what he believes.

—Anton Chekhov

In the preceding chapters of this book I have stressed the importance of the mind/body connection. I have talked about how ensuring the health of your body can protect the health of your brain, I've explained how underlying physical conditions can have negative effects on your mental health, and I have provided you with nutritional and lifestyle strategies that enhance and protect the interrelationship between good physical health and good brain health. I hope you see clearly that the ways in which you treat your body can positively influence the health of your brain. Now I want to talk to you about the other side of the coin: how your brain can have a dramatic impact on your body's health.

In the beginning of this book, I challenged you to be part of a paradigm shift in defining the concept of successful aging and in quality of life as we grow older. What I want to leave you with is my thoughts on another, equally potent, paradigm that is emerging.

Psychoneuroimmunology (PNI) is the scientific study of the interconnections between the body's most complex systems—the emotions, the brain, and the immune system. My interest in psychoneuroimmunology and its applications for optimal health was sparked by a 1973 study conducted at Johns Hopkins University.[1] This study reported the discovery of receptors on our immune cells for neuropeptides. Neuropeptides are chemicals produced by the brain that fluctuate according to our emotions. The results of this study indicate that a person's immune system is affected by a person's thoughts. In essence, how you think you feel is how you feel.

This scientific discovery reaffirms my personal philosophy that there is no more important force in human history than belief. Jesus, Mohammad, Moses, Buddha, Copernicus, Mother Teresa, Martin Luther King Jr., Thomas Edison, and Winston Churchill—all of these great historical figures had an unshakable belief system as their anchor.

We all have heard about individuals experiencing dramatic improvements in their health as a result of taking a placebo. Many attribute the positive effects of placebos to psychological forces—a strong belief that the treatment will work, or a feeling that it is working. Irving Kirsch, a psychologist at the University of Connecticut, attributes the effectiveness of Prozac and other drugs almost entirely to the placebo effect. Kirsch conducted an experiment in which he analyzed nineteen clinical trials of antidepressants, concluding that the belief in improvement of the condition, as opposed to the alterations in brain chemistry, was responsible for 75 percent of the drugs' effectiveness.[2]

There are studies that indicate the existence of a circuit that connects the immune system and the brain—connecting illness or stress and thought. Traditional medicine has dismissed the notion that going outside in the cold can result in one catching a cold; nonetheless, there is much anecdotal evidence that contradicts this belief. New research is on the horizon that may make those "old wives' tales" (as described by those who discount this anecdotal evidence) accepted by traditional medicine.

Steven Maier, Ph.D., a University of Colorado Distinguished Professor and the Director of the Center for Neuroscience, has explored two broad areas of research in the connection between stress and immunity functions. Dr. Maier studies the manner in which the brain regulates the immune system *and* how immune system cells send signals to the brain. The primary focus of his studies concerns comprehending the mechanisms of immune-to-brain signaling at various levels.[3]

The other major area of Dr. Maier's study concerns the variables that regulate the impact stressors have on brain chemistry and the neurochemical mechanisms that allow these stressors to change behavior, mood, and the organism's reactions to drugs.[4] This aspect of the study is primarily concerned with the degree to which behavioral control organisms are able to exercise control over stressors. The research indicates that stress—perhaps even the stress of being cold—appears to connect to the same immune system–nervous system mechanism that ignites common cold symptoms.

For more than a decade, researchers have known that behavioral and psychological events can influence the immune system. What the study of psychoneuroimmunology tells us is that our beliefs cannot only change our perception of reality, but they can also change reality itself. In a remarkable case study, a woman in California had a cancerous tumor, so bad that it was described as resembling "a hand grenade under a thin sheathing of skin." Her doctors, who had suggested she have a mastectomy, sent her to an alternative physician, who assisted her in visualization. One of the exercises involved increasing her body temperature. During this exercise, the temperature of her skin rose by 14 degrees. The woman responded extremely well to this treatment, and upon her return to her primary doctors two weeks later, it was found that the tumor had completely disappeared.[5]

In another study, researchers found that rheumatoid arthritis seemed to be connected to the strength of the individual's psychological defenses. Those patients with weakened psychological defenses were more liable to have rapidly developing cases of the disease, respond poorly to treatment, and become incapacitated.[6]

Maier's research is particularly interested in the knee-jerk reaction of our immune system, which determines whether we become ill as a result of certain stressors. This nonspecific immune response is frequently referred to as the "sickness" response. When activated, it sets in motion a series of physiological and behavioral changes, like fever, alterations in the liver's metabolism, decreased consumption of food and liquid, and decreased sexual desire. This nonspecific immune response also triggers the classic response to stress—commonly referred to as fight or flight—the release of stress-fighting hormones, including cortisol.

Maier believes that the sickness pattern is an organized effort on the part of the body, designed to manufacture energy to fight infection and to preserve energy. Maier and his colleagues determined the molecules called proinflammatory cytokines—interleukin-1, interleukin-6, and tumor necrosis factor alpha—were signaling the brain.[7]

When Maier inactivated these cytokines or blocked the cerebral receptors that connect them, animals did not show any indication that they were sick following infection. When these cytokines were activated, however, the animals exhibited all of the classic signs of infection, whether they were sick or not.

Interestingly enough, Maier discovered that it is not the cytokines manufactured in the blood that signal to the brain that you are sick. Remember the blood-brain barrier? The cytokines are too big to get past it. Instead, when infection–fighting cells called macrophages attack a bacteria, a cytokine called interleukin-1 is released into the bloodstream, where it binds to receptors on the paraganglia—cells found near the adrenal glands that release the neurotransmitters epinephrine and norepinephrine. These neurotransmitters activate the brain's vagus nerve, which controls the functions of the larynx, stomach, esophagus, heart, lungs, and intestines. This signal triggers the brain to make its own cytokines, setting off the sickness response, which then signals back to the immune system and further activates immune cells. Maier calls this loop from infection-fighting blood cells to cranial nerves to a systemic immune reaction "complete biodirectional immune-to-brain circuitry."

In addition to this chemical brain–immune system response, Maier discovered that if animals were stressed—by socially isolating them or giving them electrical shock—their brains would produce massive increases in the cytokine interleukin-1 in the hippocampus.[8] Along with the predicted stress response, the animals exhibited behavioral and physiological changes—a decrease in food and water consumption, fever, increased white blood cell count, and activated macrophages—just like those seen in the infection-driven "sickness" response.[9]

The implications of this shared neural loop are that stress and infection sensitize the body's reaction to the other. In other words, an infection primes the circuit so that it has an exaggerated response to later stress, and vice versa. According to Maier, "Stress is another form of infection. And the consequences of stress are mediated by the activation of circuits that actually evolved to defend against infection."[10]

For many years the concept of mind/body interactions has been discounted by traditional medicine. When scientific research demonstrates an example of such a connection, it is often dismissed by the traditional medical community as a placebo effect. Yet the mind/body connection has been proven by the tens of thousands of drug studies that employ the traditionally accepted double-blind, placebo-controlled method.

It is one thing for Deepak Chopra, Adele Davis, Carlton Fredericks, myself, or any other alternative medicine practitioners to state their belief in the mind/body connection, but it took a well-respected member of the orthodox medical community to give it mainstream credibility. In 1974, Dr. Herbert Benson and his colleagues pioneered the discovery of the relaxation response, and a year later published the seminal work on the subject, entitled *The Relaxation Response*.[11] Based on studies at Boston's Beth Israel Hospital and Harvard Medical School, Dr. Benson showed that relaxation techniques such as meditation have immense physical benefits and are effective in treating such disparate conditions as hypertension, heart disease, and cancer. This book ushered in a new era in the study of the mind/body connection.

In 1993, the field and concept of mind/body medicine were brought into the homes of mainstream America by one of its most respected journalists when Bill Moyers hosted his PBS television special entitled *Healing and the Mind*. Throughout the series, Moyers explored the uncharted waters of the mind/body connection through a series of interviews with acclaimed experts, as well as ordinary laypersons. The author showed the American public for the first time how the new innovations in the mind/body field were being used to treat stress, chronic disease, and neonatal problems in hospitals throughout America. Moyers also delved into the chemical connection of emotions and their ability to either make us well or make us sick.

Later, experiments conducted by the well-respected Dr. Andrew Weil confirmed that the benefit of a treatment almost always mirrored the expectations of the patient. In one amazing case, reported in his book *Spontaneous Healing*,[12] a woman with advanced lupus and kidney failure was in failing health when she fell in love. Shortly thereafter, her symptoms disappeared. Dr. Weil reported that the remarkable shift in her level of consciousness coincided precisely with the full remission of her disease. The power of her mind, her beliefs, and her attitude was accepted as positively impacting her medical condition.

But this field did not just arrive in the 1970s or 1980s. It merely took that long for it to be *accepted* by the mainstream. Thirty years ago the medical establishment laughed at me for stating that simply by changing one's lifestyle a person's health could be improved. They are not laughing at me today. Virtually every day I see a new report touting the benefits of lifestyle change in combating a wide array of conditions. Just a sampling of the spate of recent reports shows how brain exercise is the key to a healthy mind,[13] that lifestyle plays a significant role in Alzheimer's disease,[14] and that lifestyle is crucial in combating diabetes.[15]

In order to properly understand the use of mind/body medicine, one must place it in its proper context. Lifestyle changes designed to improve the health of the individual must occur first, for the mind/body techniques are only one of many areas of lifestyle change that synergistically improve health. Recent medical studies confirm that proper diet, exercise, and social support networks are integral pieces of this puzzle.

We all have had the experience of being involved in an extremely stressful situation—an argument with a loved one, the death of a close friend, being fired from one's job—and shortly thereafter coming down with a cold, or just feeling miserable. Up until relatively recently, there was no scientific support establishing a relationship between the two. The thought that feelings could adversely affect physical health was an alien one to the medical community.

But a plethora of scientific evidence has now established a definite link between feelings and physical health. This evidence demonstrates how the brain regulates the immune system—the body's main guardian against infectious diseases—in extremely complex and critical ways by sending a steady barrage of messages to it. As we have seen, however, this is a two-way street, for the brain also receives messages from the immune system.

In all of the cases I've used as illustrations in this chapter, the single constant in successful outcomes was the belief of the individual. This belief was relayed to the brain, to the immune system, or to the nervous system. Once this belief was firmly entrenched, the body and brain went into action and performed miracles.

One of my favorite examples of the power of the mind to control the body is that of the runner Roger Bannister. Up until 1954, it was widely believed that humans were incapable of running the mile in under four minutes. It was thought that it was physically impossible for a person to do so. Then Roger Bannister ran the mile in 3:59:4. Less than six weeks after Bannister broke the record, John Landy from Australia lowered the record by another second. And, within the next nine years, nearly two hundred people had broken the "impossible" barrier. Now, high school athletes routinely break it. Bannister demonstrated that the barrier was purely psychological. But the significant aspect to this story is that any of those two hundred people could have figured it out on their own. They didn't really need Bannister to show them the fallacy of this belief.

The four-minute mile is a metaphor for life. It is a metaphor for everything that everyone has told you that you could not do. But now you have the knowledge to prove them wrong. Your health is in your hands and in your mind.

CHAPTER 15

MIND POWER MEALS

RECIPES FOR THE MIND

The late comedian Redd Foxx used to joke, "They say you are what you eat. No wonder you look like garbage to me." Truer words were never spoken. You not only literally become what you eat, but what you eat determines how you think, what kind of mood you are in, how you feel, and your emotional stability. Furthermore, it has been proven that what you eat can increase your IQ, enhance your memory, and reverse the aging process.

Through my extensive travels, I have noticed that the vast majority of individuals I meet are nowhere near maximizing their brains' full potential in terms of intelligence, focusing, and memory. Little do they know that with the proper types and amounts of nutrients, they could drastically improve their overall health and brain function.

It is important to consume foods as they were grown in nature. Organic fresh fruits and vegetables, whole grains, legumes, nuts and seeds, and (for those who are not vegetarians) nontoxic animal proteins head the list. Purchase organic foods that have not been exposed to pesticides or other chemical sprays and are not packed with additives.

Eating right does not have to involve a huge effort. Prepare healthy dishes in larger quantities and store them for use throughout the week.

The following recipes were created specifically to promote the health and vitality of your brain. Our brains are under constant assault from a variety of sources: stress, work, home life, improper relationships, free radical damage, electromagnetic radiation, improper nutrition, and so on. To gain the most benefit from my eating plan, you must be consistent in your approach and committed to the health and welfare of your brain. You cannot exercise and eat properly for a month, then take a month off. After all, cell-damaging free radicals never take a day off.

Too many people are literally digging their own graves with their forks. Why not build a temple?

RECIPES

Beverages

Antioxidant Punch
Antioxidant Supreme
Apple Pear Gingerale
Apple Sprouts
The Big Cleanse
Blueberry and Pear Macadamia Nut Shake
Brain Juice
Brain Power
Carrot, Pineapple, and Strawberry Juice
Chilling Relaxer
Chlorophyll Boost
Cucumber Coolade
Deep Sea Juicing
Delicious Detox
Detox Tonic
Enzyme Enhancer
Everglades Punch
Fatigue Buster
Flax Cruncher
Fountain of Youth
Free Radical Delight
Gary's Gingerale
Gingermint Tea
Green Power Punch
Head Cleaner
How Green Is Your Juice

The Kitchen Sink
Melon Boost
Nuts and Seeds
Pure Citrus Punch
Relax Your Mind
Ruby Red
Sleep Insurer
Strong Lungs
Super Vegetable Cocktail
Velvety Pecan Milk
Wisdom Drink

Salads

Fabulous Wild Rice Salad
Four Bean Salad
Gary's Chef's Salad with Creamy Italian Dressing
Herbed Tomato Salad
Insalata Caesar
Mixed Beans Vinaigrette
Mixed Sprout, Bean, and Nut Salad with Lime Vinaigrette
Nature's Total Salad with Lemon Garlic Dressing
Pasta Salad
Succotash Salad
Superior Spinach Salad

Soups

Black Bean Soup
Chilled Cantaloupe Soup
Chinese Mushroom Soup
Cinnamon Fruit Soup
Cold Strawberry Soup
Cream of Sweet Potato Soup
Creamy Tomato Soup
Papaya Nectar Soup

Breakfast

Blueberry Breakfast Treat
Blueberry-Banana Pancakes
Blueberry Buckwheat-Soy-Banana Pancakes
Cream of Barley
Nutty Banana Breakfast
Nutty Oatmeal
Rice and Strawberries

Main Dishes

Brazilian Rice
Chickpea Hummus with Toasted Pita Triangles
Gary's Vegetable Pan
Gary's Veggieball Stew
Good Shepherd's Pie
Indonesian Kale
Italian Vegetable Stew
Macaroni Marconi
Original Broccoli Stir-Fry
Pasta Fagioli (Bean Soup)
Potato Chowder
Ratatouille
Sweet Kidney Bean Mash
Tantalizing Tempeh Dinner
Tex-Mex Tofu Scrambler

Desserts

Blackberry Nectarine Fruit Salad
Carob Power Brownies
Cherry Grape Kanten
Cold Cherry Soup
Heavenly Roasted Nuts

Beverages

ANTIOXIDANT PUNCH

1 pineapple, peeled, cored, and cut into 1-inch cubes
4 large limes, peeled and quartered
2 cups unsweetened cranberry juice
1 cup concord grape juice
24 ice cubes
1 large lime, sliced into ½-inch-thick half-moons (for garnish)
2 pineapple wedges, sliced into ½-inch-thick fans (for garnish)

Separately juice pineapple and limes. In a large pitcher or punch bowl, combine the pineapple and lime juices with the cranberry juice, grape juice, and ice. Stir together until well combined. Serve garnished with lime and pineapple slices.

ANTIOXIDANT SUPREME

½ honeydew, cubed (do not remove skin)
15 grapes (do not use seedless grapes)
½ cup organic red wine (no sulfites), preferably nonalcoholic
2 T aloe vera concentrate

Juice honeydew and grapes. Blend the juices with wine and aloe vera concentrate in a container.

APPLE PEAR GINGERALE

1 large apple, cored and quartered   *2 cups sparkling mineral water*
1 large pear, cored and quartered   *6 ice cubes*
1 ounce fresh ginger, sliced into
*   ½-inch pieces*

Juice apple, pear, and ginger. In a large pitcher, combine the apple juice mixture and mineral water. Stir together until well combined. Serve over ice.

APPLE SPROUTS

4 apples, cored and quartered
2 yams, cubed
1 cup alfalfa sprouts

Separately juice the ingredients. Combine the juices and serve immediately.

THE BIG CLEANSE

½ clove organic garlic, peeled
2 cups collard greens, chopped
2 cups organic cauliflower, chopped
½ cup red beet, cubed
1 cup organic chard, chopped
2 large apples, cored and quartered
2 ounces wheatgrass juice

Separately juice the garlic, collard greens, cauliflower, red beet, chard, and apples. Combine the juices and add the wheatgrass juice. Stir well.

(Wheatgrass can be juiced by using a wheatgrass press. You can also make wheatgrass juice by squeezing the grass into clusters with your hand and juicing these hand-squeezed wheatgrass clusters through a traditional fruit and vegetable juicer.)

BLUEBERRY AND PEAR MACADAMIA NUT SHAKE

2 pears (½ cup juice)
½ cup blueberries
½ cup ground or whole white
  macadamia nuts, unsalted

1 banana, mashed
½ cup unsweetened rice milk
2 heaping T protein powder
½ tsp pure lemon extract

Juice pears. In a blender, combine pear juice with the blueberries, macadamia nuts, mashed banana, rice milk, protein powder, and lemon extract. Blend for 2 minutes, or until smooth. Serve immediately.

BRAIN JUICE

1½ cups organic green beans
½ head organic cabbage, shredded
2 cups organic collard greens, chopped
1 cup organic spinach
2 medium organic peaches, quartered and pitted
3 oranges, peeled and quartered

Separately juice the green beans, cabbage, collard greens, spinach, peaches, and oranges. Combine the juices and serve immediately.

BRAIN POWER

12 leechi nuts (pitted)
2 oranges, quartered
2 mangoes, diced and pitted
100 mg ginseng
100 mg ginkgo biloba

Remove seeds and skin from the leechi nuts. Separately juice the leechi nuts, oranges, and mangoes. In a blender or food processor, combine the juices with the herbs and blend until smooth.

CARROT, PINEAPPLE, AND STRAWBERRY JUICE

1 cup of strawberries, halved
4 carrots, sliced
½ pineapple, cubed and peeled

Remove stems or leaves from strawberries. Separately juice the strawberries, carrots, and pineapple. Combine the juices and serve immediately.

CHILLING RELAXER

½ pint organic dandelion flowers and stems
2 pints medium organic strawberries
1 medium piece organic cantaloupe (peeled)
2 T organic flax oil
2 ounces organic wheatgrass juice
1 T lecithin

Separately juice the dandelions, strawberries, and cantaloupe. Combine juices and add flax oil, wheatgrass juice, and lecithin. Stir well.

(Wheatgrass juice can be made by using a wheatgrass press. You can also make wheatgrass juice by squeezing the grass into clusters with your hand and juicing these hand-squeezed wheatgrass clusters through a traditional fruit and vegetable juicer.)

CHLOROPHYLL BOOST

2 cups organic alfalfa sprouts
2 cups organic spinach, chopped
2 cups organic collard greens, chopped (ends cut)
5 medium stalks organic asparagus
2 ounces wheatgrass juice
1 apple (optional), cored and quartered

Separately juice the alfalfa sprouts, spinach, collard greens, and asparagus, and combine with the wheatgrass juice. Juice an apple and add the juice to the mixture if you find the greens alone to be too bitter.

(Wheatgrass juice can be made by using a wheatgrass press. You can also make wheatgrass juice by squeezing the grass into clusters with your hand and juicing these hand-squeezed wheatgrass clusters through a traditional fruit and vegetable juicer.)

CRANBERRY COOLER

4 cups filtered water
2 green tea bags (decaffeinated)
4 large oranges, peeled
2 large limes, peeled
1 large lemon, peeled
1 cup unsweetened cranberry juice
2 cups blueberries
¼ cup honey
1 tsp ground cinnamon
20 ice cubes
1 large lime, sliced into ½-inch-thick half-moons (for garnish)

In a small saucepan with lid, combine the water and tea bags, bring to a boil, then simmer covered for 8–10 minutes, or until fully brewed. Set aside to cool completely. Separately juice the oranges, limes, and lemon. In a blender, combine the juices with the cranberry juice, blueberries, honey, cinnamon, ice cubes, and tea. Blend on high speed for 3 minutes or until well combined. Serve over ice and garnish with lime slices.

CUCUMBER COOLADE

1 large bunch flat-leaf parsley
4 large cucumbers, cut into quarters lengthwise
4 pears, cored and quartered
1 small piece ginger (1 inch square)

Bunch up the parsley and push it through the juicer feed tube, alternating it with the cucumbers, pears, and ginger. Serve immediately.

DEEP SEA JUICING

1 ounce wakame sea vegetable
1 ounce kombu sea vegetable
1 ounce dulse sea vegetables
2 cups arugula lettuce, chopped
2 cups organic red leaf lettuce, chopped
2 cups organic romaine lettuce, chopped
2 apples, cored and quartered

Cut the wakame, kombu, and dulse into small pieces and chop very fine in blender or food processor. Separately juice the arugula, red leaf, and romaine lettuces, and the apples. Add the juices to the vegetables in the blender or food processor and blend until well combined. Serve immediately.

DELICIOUS DETOX

½ small watermelon, cubed (do not remove rind)
2 cups frozen cherries (pitted)
2 cups alfalfa sprouts
½ pint blueberries
½ pint raspberries
1 medium organic peach, pitted and quartered

Separately juice the watermelon, cherries, alfalfa sprouts, blueberries, raspberries, and peach. Combine the juices and serve immediately.

DETOX TONIC

1 watermelon, cubed (do not remove rind)
8 kiwifruit, peeled
2 grapefruits, peeled and quartered
2 limes, peeled and quartered
1 lemon, peeled and quartered

Push the watermelon, kiwifruit, grapefruits, limes, and lemon through the juicer feed tube. Serve immediately.

ENZYME ENHANCER

1 medium organic papaya, cubed
½ large organic pineapple, cubed and peeled
6–10 large organic strawberries, halved, with stems and leaves removed
½ medium organic cabbage, chopped
½ small organic kiwi, quartered

Separately juice the papaya, pineapple, strawberries, cabbage, and kiwi. Combine the juices and serve immediately.

EVERGLADES PUNCH

1 honeydew melon, peeled, seeded, and cut into 2-inch pieces (about 8 cups)
4 large oranges, peeled and quartered
4 large limes, peeled and quartered
2 large grapefruits, peeled and quartered
2 large lemons, peeled and quartered
4 mangoes, peeled, pitted, and cut into 2-inch pieces
1 cup blueberries
20–40 ice cubes
1 large orange, sliced into ½-inch-thick half-moons (for garnish)

Push the melon, oranges, limes, grapefruits, lemons, mangoes, and blueberries through the juicer feed tube. Serve over ice and garnish with orange slices.

FATIGUE BUSTER

3 carrots, sliced lengthwise   *1 pear, cored and quartered*
2 cucumbers, sliced   *½ tsp bee propolis*

Separately juice the carrots, cucumbers, and pear. Combine the juices and stir in the bee propolis. Serve immediately.

(If allergic to bee propolis, replace with ½ tsp guarana or ginseng powder. Powders can be removed from capsules.)

FLAX CRUNCHER

3 T organic flax seed
1 cup organic puffed rice
1 cup tofu yogurt
½ cup Rice Dream Original

In a grinder, grind the flax seed very fine. In a blender, chop the puffed rice. Add the flax seed, tofu yogurt, and Rice Dream to the chopped puffed rice and blend well.

FOUNTAIN OF YOUTH

1 cup green grapes
1 cup purple grapes
½ cantaloupe, cubed and peeled
2 medium organic zucchini, sliced
1 medium tomato, quartered
2 T vegetarian protein powder

Separately juice the green and purple grapes, cantaloupe, zucchini, and tomato. In a blender, combine the juices with the protein powder and blend well.

FREE RADICAL DELIGHT

1 cup organic grapes
½ medium organic cantaloupe, cubed and peeled
½ cup organic broccoli, chopped
1 cup organic collard greens, chopped (ends cut)
1 cup organic spinach, chopped (ends cut)
3 oranges, quartered

Separately juice the grapes, cantaloupe, broccoli, collard greens, spinach, and oranges. Combine the juices and serve immediately.

GARY'S GINGERALE

organic ginger, 1-inch piece
½ large organic cantaloupe, cubed (do not remove rind)
½ pint organic strawberries, halved and stemmed
1 medium organic orange, quartered (do not remove peel)
4 ounces sparkling water

Separately juice the ginger, cantaloupe, strawberries, and orange. Combine the juices and add the sparkling water. Serve immediately.

GINGERMINT TEA

8 cups filtered water
4 peppermint tea bags
  (decaffeinated)
4 ounces fresh ginger, sliced into
  ½-inch pieces
1 T plus 1 tsp honey (optional)

½ cup freshly squeezed lemon juice
40 ice cubes
1 large lemon, sliced into
  ½-inch-thick half-moons
  (for garnish)
fresh mint (optional)

In a small saucepan with a lid, combine the water, tea bags, and ginger over moderate heat and simmer covered for 8–10 minutes, or until fully brewed. Sir in the honey until well combined and set aside to cool completely. Combine the tea, lemon juice, and ice in a large pitcher. Stir together. Serve garnished with lemon slices and fresh mint.

GREEN POWER PUNCH

2 cups kale, chopped
2 cups organic parsley, chopped
1 cup organic spinach, chopped
1 medium organic apple, cored and
  quartered

1 cup broccoli, chopped
½ head cauliflower, chopped
6 stalks celery

Separately juice kale, parsley, spinach, apple, broccoli, cauliflower, and celery. Combine juices and serve immediately.

HEAD CLEANER

1 small onion, quartered and peeled
3 cloves garlic, peeled
2 stalks celery
1 turnip, halved (do not remove leaves)
ginger, ½-inch slice
3 T honey

Separately juice onion, garlic, celery, turnip, and ginger. Combine juices and add honey. Stir well.

HOW GREEN IS YOUR JUICE

2 cups kale, chopped
2 cups spinach, chopped
2 stalks celery
2 tsp green vegetable powder (available at most health food stores)

Separately juice the kale, spinach, and celery. In a blender, combine the juices with the green vegetable powder and blend well. Serve immediately.

THE KITCHEN SINK

1 apple, cored and quartered
1 cup spinach, chopped
1 cup kale, chopped
½ cup chard, chopped
½ papaya, cubed
2 cloves garlic, peeled
organic ginger, ½-inch piece
2 T protein powder

Separately juice apple, spinach, kale, chard, papaya, garlic, and ginger. In a blender, combine juices and protein powder and mix well.

MELON BOOST

½ medium cantaloupe, peeled and cubed
½ small watermelon (without rind), cubed
1 medium lemon, peeled and quartered
½ tsp vitamin C powder
1 pint raspberries

Separately juice cantaloupe, watermelon, and lemon. In a blender, combine the juices, vitamin C powder, and raspberries, and mix well.

NUTS AND SEEDS

2½ cups vanilla soy milk
1 pint blueberries
2 frozen bananas, peeled
3 T organic soy butter
3 T organic almond butter
3 T organic cashew butter
3 T organic macadamia butter
3 T organic sunflower butter

In a blender, combine soy milk, blueberries, and bananas. Add the butters and blend until smooth. Serve immediately.

PURE CITRUS PUNCH

8 large grapefruits, peeled and cubed
12 large oranges, peeled and cubed
8 large limes, peeled and quartered
4 large lemons, peeled and quartered
16–20 ice cubes

Separately juice the grapefruits, oranges, limes, and lemons. Combine the juices and serve over ice.

RELAX YOUR MIND

4 stalks celery
3 carrots, sliced lengthwise
2 apples, cored and quartered
ginger, 1-inch piece
kava kava (1 capsule/25 mg)
chamomile (1 capsule/25 mg)
St. John's wort (1 capsule/100 mg)
valerian (1 capsule/50 mg)
½ tsp nutmeg
½ tsp cinnamon

Separately juice celery, carrots, apples, and ginger. In a blender, combine juices, and empty the powder from the capsules into the liquid. Add nutmeg and cinnamon, and mix well.

RUBY RED

1 grapefruit, peeled and quartered
1 pear, cored and quartered
½ cup strawberries
½ cup blueberries
1 tsp lecithin
½ cup ice

In a blender, combine grapefruit, pear, strawberries, blueberries, and lecithin with ice and blend until smooth.

SLEEP INSURER

organic ginger root, 1-inch piece
½ cup organic basil
1 cup green beans
3 stalks organic celery
½ head cabbage, chopped
2 medium organic bananas
valerian root extract

Separately juice the ginger, basil, green beans, celery, and cabbage. In a blender, combine juices and bananas. Add 10–15 drops liquid valerian root and blend until smooth.

STRONG LUNGS

6 large organic carrots, sliced lengthwise
1 organic apple, cored and quartered
1 organic avocado, peeled, quartered, and pitted
½ large guava fruit, peeled, seeded, and quartered
3 tsp liquid chlorophyll

Separately juice the carrots, apple, avocado, and guava fruit. Combine the juices and add liquid chlorophyll. Stir well.

SUPER VEGETABLE COCKTAIL

1 large bunch flat-leaf parsley (about ½ pound)
2 large tomatoes, cored and quartered
8 large celery stalks
4 large carrots, tops removed and cut into halves lengthwise
4 yellow bell peppers, cored, seeded, and cut into quarters
4 large limes, peeled
sea salt to taste (about ½ tsp)
4 celery stalks (for garnish)
1 large lime, sliced into ½-inch-thick half-moons (for garnish)

Separately juice the parsley, then alternate pushing the tomatoes, celery, carrots, peppers, and limes through the juicer tube. Stir in salt until well combined. Serve garnished with celery stalks and lime slices.

VELVETY PECAN MILK

1 cup pecan halves, soaked in 4 cups filtered water for 6–8 hours
  (then discard soaking water, rinse well, and drain)
4 cups filtered water
2 T honey
1 T pure almond flavor
2 T pure vanilla flavor
1 pinch salt

Combine the prepared pecans and 4 cups water in a blender. Blend on medium speed for 30 seconds; increase speed to high, and continue blending for 1 minute.

Transfer the pecan mixture to a cheesecloth-lined fine sieve and strain into a medium-size bowl (squeeze or use a spoon to stir and push the milk through while you pour, since it will be too rich to strain it through without a bit of mashing). Save the pulp for hot cereal, grain dishes, baked goods, or smoothies.

Rinse and dry the blender, then pour in the strained milk, honey, almond flavor, vanilla flavor, and salt. Blend on high speed until smooth and frothy, about 1 minute. Transfer to a container and refrigerate for 1–2 hours or until chilled.

WISDOM DRINK

3 burdock roots, sliced
2 parsnips, sliced
4 carrots, sliced lengthwise
1 cup parsley greens
1 T blackstrap molasses

Separately juice the burdock, parsnips, carrots, and parsley greens. In a blender, combine juices and add molasses. Blend well and serve immediately.

Salads

FABULOUS WILD RICE SALAD

3 cups cooked wild rice
½ cup carrots, sliced
½ cup broccoli florets, steamed 5–6 minutes
½ cup fresh parsley, chopped
½ cup zucchini, diced
3 T safflower oil
1 tsp fresh dill, chopped
2 T fresh lemon juice
½ tsp freshly ground black pepper
½ tsp salt

Combine all the ingredients in a medium-size bowl, mix well, toss, and serve at room temperature.

FOUR BEAN SALAD

½ cup dry chickpeas
½ cup dry black beans
½ cup dry kidney beans
½ pound fresh string beans, cut
* into 1-inch pieces*
1–2 carrots, grated

3 scallions, sliced
½ green pepper, chopped
1 large celery stalk, diced or
* chopped*
Orange Vinaigrette (see below)

Soak the chickpeas, the black beans, and the kidney beans in separate pots of water, covered, overnight. Drain. Add unsalted water to each pot and cook the soaked beans, covered, for about an hour, or until tender. Drain, put into separate containers, and refrigerate until chilled. Steam the string beans for 5 minutes, or until just tender. Place in the refrigerator to chill. In a large mixing bowl, combine the chilled beans and the vegetables. Pour Orange Vinaigrette over the mixture and refrigerate several hours, or overnight. Serve on a bed of lettuce topped with some grated nondairy cheddar cheese, or use this salad to stuff a pita along with the nondairy cheese slices.

ORANGE VINAIGRETTE

1 tsp orange zest, minced
1 pint fresh orange juice
2 T apple cider vinegar
½ sweet onion
2 T of honey
1 garlic clove, finely chopped
1 tsp cumin seed, toasted and ground
1 tsp salt
1 tsp basil
1 tsp fennel
2 T extra-virgin olive oil
1 pinch cayenne pepper
2 T apple cider vinegar
1 T kosher salt

Combine all the ingredients in a small bowl and whisk together. Blend until smooth.

GARY'S CHEF'S SALAD WITH CREAMY ITALIAN DRESSING

1 head fresh, young romaine lettuce
1 head butter lettuce (about 1½ pounds)
Creamy Italian Dressing (see page 269)
2 cups Savory Croutons (see below)
one recipe "Bacon" Bits (see page 268)
4 ounces Vidalia onion, thinly sliced
⅓ cup black olives, pitted

Trim the base of the lettuces and discard any bruised outer leaves. Use the tender inner leaves, keeping the small leaves whole and cutting or tearing the larger outer leaves crosswise into halves or thirds. Wash and dry the greens in a spinner, and transfer to a large bowl. Drizzle the dressing onto the salad greens to taste, and gently toss together until well coated. Toss briefly with the croutons, "Bacon" Bits, onion, and olives, and serve immediately.

SAVORY CROUTONS

2 cups millet or rice bread, cut into ¾-inch cubes
2 T extra-virgin olive oil
1 T grated Parmesan-style nondairy cheese
½ tsp dried basil
½ tsp dried marjoram
½ tsp dried oregano
sea salt to taste

Preheat the oven to 425°F. Line an 11-×-15-inch cookie sheet with parchment paper and set aside. In a medium mixing bowl, toss together the bread, oil, cheese, basil, marjoram, oregano, and salt. Evenly spread the seasoned cubes on the prepared cookie sheet, and bake in the preheated oven for 8–10 minutes, or until golden. For uniformity in baking, rotate the sheet from front to back halfway through the baking period. Remove the sheet from the oven and cool the croutons completely.

"BACON" BITS

1 pound extra-firm tofu, crumbled
½ cup extra-virgin olive oil
1 large clove garlic, peeled and finely chopped
1 tsp dried marjoram
1 tsp rubbed sage
1 tsp dried basil
½ tsp dried oregano
½ tsp sea salt
freshly ground black pepper to taste (optional)

Preheat the broiler. Line an 11-×-15-inch cookie sheet with parchment paper and set aside. In a medium mixing bowl, toss together the tofu, oil, garlic, marjoram, sage, basil, oregano, salt, and pepper. Evenly spread the seasoned tofu on the prepared cookie sheet, and broil in the preheated oven for 15 minutes, or until golden. For uniformity in broiling, rotate the sheet from front to back halfway through the baking period. Remove the sheet from the oven and cool the bits completely.

CREAMY ITALIAN DRESSING

1 cup silken tofu
½ cup extra-virgin olive oil
½ cup freshly squeezed lemon juice (about 2 large lemons)
½ cup parsley, chopped
2 large cloves garlic, peeled and finely chopped
16 fresh basil leaves
½ tsp sea salt
freshly ground black pepper to taste (optional)

In a blender, combine the tofu, oil, lemon juice, parsley, garlic, basil, salt, and pepper. Blend on medium speed for 3 minutes, or until smooth and creamy. Set aside.

HERBED TOMATO SALAD

1 tsp sea salt
⅛ tsp cayenne pepper
½ tsp freshly ground black pepper
2 T lime juice
2 T fresh dill
½ tsp chopped fresh thyme
3 ripe tomatoes
1 bunch arugula
1 bunch watercress

In a small bowl, combine salt, cayenne and black pepper, lime juice, dill, and thyme. Cut tomatoes into thick slices; toss with arugula and watercress. Pour dressing over salad, and let marinate for 1 hour in the refrigerator. Serve chilled.

INSALATA CAESAR

2 heads fresh, young romaine lettuce (about 1½ pounds)
Creamy Caesar Dressing (see below)
2 cups Savory Croutons (see page 268)
4 sheets julienne strips of sushi nori

Trim the base of the romaine lettuce and discard any bruised outer leaves. Use the tender inner leaves, keeping the small leaves whole and cutting or tearing the larger outer leaves crosswise into halves or thirds. Wash and dry the greens in a spinner, and transfer to a large bowl. Drizzle the dressing onto the salad greens to taste, and gently toss together until well coated. Toss briefly with the croutons, top with nori, and serve immediately.

CREAMY CAESAR DRESSING

½ cup extra-virgin olive oil
½ cup water
½ cup tahini
½ cup silken tofu
½ cup freshly squeezed lemon juice (about 1 large lemon)
1 tsp tamari soy sauce
2 T chopped parsley
1 large clove garlic, peeled and finely chopped
½ tsp dried basil
½ tsp paprika
½ tsp sea salt

In a blender, combine the oil, water, tahini, tofu, lemon juice, soy sauce, parsley, garlic, basil, paprika, and salt. Blend on medium speed for 3 minutes, or until smooth and creamy, and set aside.

MIXED BEANS VINAIGRETTE

½ cup cooked lima beans
½ cup canned kidney beans, drained
½ cup green beans, steamed 15 minutes
½ cup chopped yellow bell pepper
½ cup chopped fresh parsley
1 to 2 T prepared mustard
1 to 2 T apple cider vinegar
2 T extra-virgin olive oil
½ tsp freshly ground black pepper
2 T chopped red onions

Combine all the ingredients in a medium-size bowl, toss, and serve chilled.

MIXED SPROUT, BEAN, AND NUT SALAD WITH LIME VINAIGRETTE

2 cups sunflower sprouts
2 cups alfalfa sprouts
½ cup radish sprouts
½ cup canned garbanzo beans
½ cup asparagus tips, steamed 8–10 minutes
½ cup avocado cubes
½ cup halved seedless grapes
½ cup chopped Brazil nuts
Lime Vinaigrette (see below)

Combine all the ingredients except Lime Vinaigrette in a large salad bowl and chill for 1 hour. Serve with Lime Vinaigrette.

LIME VINAIGRETTE

¼ cup lime juice
¼ cup fresh orange juice
¼ cup raw honey
¼ cup orange zest
2 T Dijon mustard
⅛ cup agave
juice from ¼ lemon
1 cup plus 2 tsp light extra-virgin olive oil
1 T kosher salt
2 T mint
pinch tarragon seed
pinch white pepper

Place lime juice, orange juice, honey, orange zest, mustard, agave, and lemon juice in a large bowl. While blending ingredients with a whisk in one hand, slowly add the oil. Season with salt, mint, tarragon seed, and white pepper, to taste.

NATURE'S TOTAL SALAD WITH LEMON GARLIC DRESSING

2 heads fresh, young romaine lettuce (about 1½ pounds)
½ pound sunflower sprouts
Lemon Garlic Dressing (see below)
2 ripe Haas avocados, peeled, halved, pitted, and sliced
1 large cucumber, halved, seeded, and thinly sliced
1 cup cooked millet
½ cup unsalted roasted cashews

Trim the base of the lettuces and discard any bruised outer leaves. Use the tender inner leaves, keeping the small leaves whole and cutting or tearing the larger outer leaves crosswise into halves or thirds. Wash and dry the greens and sunflower sprouts in a spinner, and transfer to a large bowl. Drizzle the dressing onto the lettuce, add the sprouts, avocados, cucumber, and millet to taste, and gently toss together until well coated. Toss briefly with the cashews and serve immediately.

LEMON GARLIC DRESSING

½ cup extra-virgin olive oil
½ cup freshly squeezed lemon juice (about 2 large lemons)
1 cup parsley, chopped
2 large cloves garlic, peeled and finely chopped
2 tsp sea salt
freshly ground black pepper to taste (optional)

In a blender, combine the oil, lemon juice, parsley, garlic, salt, and pepper. Blend on medium speed for 3 minutes, or until emulsified.

PASTA SALAD

4 ounces whole wheat macaroni swirls, uncooked
1 cup soy cheese
½ tsp dry mustard
2–3 T plain soy yogurt
1 red bell pepper, coarsely chopped
4 scallions, chopped
1 T parsley flakes
1 tsp dill
1 tsp tamari (soy sauce)
salt and pepper to taste

Cook the macaroni according to the directions on the package. Drain well and chill. In a large mixing bowl, combine the soy cheese, mustard, and soy yogurt. Add the macaroni, toss well, and add the remaining ingredients. Toss again. Serve on a bed of lettuce.

SUCCOTASH SALAD

about 4 quarts filtered water
one 12-ounce package quinoa macaroni
2 large Vidalia onions, peeled and thinly sliced
½ cup extra-virgin olive oil
1 small kuri squash, seeded and chopped into ¼-inch pieces (about 2 cups)
½ pound extra-firm tofu (crumbled)
one 10-ounce package frozen lima beans
2 cups fresh corn kernels (about 3–4 ears)
one 6-ounce can pitted black olives, sliced
1 large red bell pepper, cored, seeded, and diced
4 large celery stalks, finely chopped
½ cup chopped parsley (curly leafed preferred)
½ cup freshly squeezed lemon juice
1 T plus 1 tsp sea salt
1 T dried basil
freshly ground black pepper to taste (optional)
sweet relish to taste
paprika to garnish

In a large pot, bring the water to a rolling boil. Stir the macaroni into the water and cook until the pasta is just tender, but not soft, about 4–5 minutes. Transfer to a colander, drain, and place in a large mixing bowl to cool. While the pasta is cooling, use a large saucepan to sauté the onions in the oil over moderate heat for 6–8 minutes, or until tender. Remove the onions from heat and gently toss into the cooked pasta until well blended. Place the kuri squash pieces on a steamer set into a large pot containing 1 inch of filtered water. Cook, covered, over moderate to high heat until the squash is tender when a fork is inserted into its center, about 8 minutes. Remove the squash from the steamer and gently toss into the macaroni and onion mixture. Add the tofu, lima beans, and corn to the steamer and cook covered for 10 minutes, or until the lima beans are hot. Remove the tofu, lima beans, and corn from the steamer and gently toss into the macaroni mixture. Add the olives, red pepper, celery, parsley, lemon juice, salt, basil, black pepper, and relish to the macaroni and gently toss together until well blended. Serve warm or chilled, garnished with a sprinkling of paprika.

SUPERIOR SPINACH SALAD

3 ounces spinach, coarsely chopped
3 ounces cauliflower florets, in bite-size pieces
3 ounces avocado, cut into bite-size pieces
3 ounces marinated artichoke hearts, cut into bite-size pieces
1½ ounces peanuts, chopped
1½ ounces shallots, chopped
1 T sunflower oil
½ tsp oregano
½ tsp sage
½ tsp salt

Combine all ingredients and mix well.

Soups

BLACK BEAN SOUP

3 T olive oil
1 onion, chopped
1 stalk celery, sliced
1½ cups black beans, washed very
* well*

3 cloves garlic
6 cups vegetable stock
1 tsp celery salt, or more to taste
2 T spelt flour
1 lemon, sliced

In a large soup pot, heat the olive oil and sauté the onion and celery until the onion is translucent and the celery is wilted, about 5 minutes. Add the black beans, garlic, and vegetable stock. Bring the mixture to a boil. Cover and simmer for 3 hours, or until the beans are very tender. Add the celery salt and the flour. (If you measure the flour into a sifter and sift it into the soup, you never have trouble dissolving it.) Remove from heat. Transfer the mixture in batches to a blender and purée. After puréeing each batch, pour the purée into a large bowl. When you have puréed the entire mixture, return it to the pot and cook until it thickens slightly, which will take about 20 minutes to a half hour. Some people like a more lemony flavor than others. Garnish the soup with the lemon slices and serve.

CHILLED CANTALOUPE SOUP

1 tsp agar flakes
2 T water
1 cup orange or tangerine juice
1 T lemon juice
2 cups diced cantaloupe
tofu sour cream for garnish

Place agar, water, and ¼ cup of orange juice in a small saucepan. Bring to a boil, reduce heat, and simmer until the agar dissolves, about 10 minutes. Place this mixture in a blender with the remaining orange or tangerine juice, the lemon juice, and the cantaloupe pieces. Blend until the mixture is puréed. Chill in the refrigerator for at least 1 hour, preferably longer. Just before serving, return the mixture to the blender for 1–2 minutes. Serve with a spoonful of tofu sour cream on top.

CHINESE MUSHROOM SOUP

½ cup chopped leeks
1 scallion, chopped
1 T sesame oil
½ tsp hot sesame oil
1 T tamari
2 cloves garlic, sliced
1½ tsp freshly grated ginger
½ cup diced firm tofu
½ cup miso paste
5 cups water

½ cup water chestnuts (measured, then chopped)
½ cup bamboo shoots (measured, then chopped)
½ cup dried black mushrooms
½ cup tree ear mushrooms
½ cup shiitake mushrooms (heads only)
1 tsp freshly ground black pepper
1 T nori flakes for garnish

In a large saucepan, sauté the leeks and scallion in the oils over medium-high heat for 5 minutes. Add the tamari, garlic, ginger, and tofu, and sauté another 3 minutes. Whisk in the miso paste and water. Add the remaining ingredients, except the nori flakes, reduce the heat to low, and let simmer for 50 minutes. Garnish with the nori flakes.

CINNAMON FRUIT SOUP

1 butternut squash (½ cup juice and ¾ cup pulp)
2 pears (½ cup juice)
1½ cups unsweetened soy milk
1 tsp pure vanilla extract
½ tsp ground cinnamon
6 orange slices (for garnish)
2 sprigs fresh mint (for garnish)

Separately juice the squash and pears to get ½ cup of squash juice, ¾ cup of squash pulp, and ½ cup of pear juice. In a medium-size saucepan, combine the juices, pulp, soy milk, vanilla extract, and cinnamon. Bring to a boil over high heat. Reduce the heat to medium-low, and simmer uncovered for 4–6 minutes. Serve hot or cold, garnished with the orange slices and mint sprigs, if desired.

COLD STRAWBERRY SOUP

1 pint strawberries, hulled
1 cup fruit juice (orange, papaya, apple, strawberry)
2 T arrowroot
juice of 1 lemon
honey to taste
½ cup tofu sour cream
tofu sour cream for garnish

Place three-quarters of the strawberries and the cup of fruit juice into a blender and purée. Pour the mixture into a saucepan. Dissolve the arrowroot in the lemon juice and pour this mixture into the saucepan as well. Cook over medium heat until the mixture thickens, about 5 minutes. Remove from heat and sweeten with honey, if desired. Slice the remaining strawberries and fold them, along with the ½ cup of tofu sour cream, into a slightly cooled mixture. Refrigerate 2–3 hours, until well chilled. Serve cold with a teaspoonful of tofu sour cream on top.

CREAM OF SWEET POTATO SOUP

2 T unsalted nondairy butter
3 cloves garlic, minced or pressed
1 large onion, thinly sliced
2 sweet potatoes (about 1 pound), sliced

2 cups low-sodium vegetable stock
1 bunch fresh watercress
2 cups soy milk
egg substitute for 2 egg yolks

In a large, heavy saucepan, melt the butter. Add the garlic and onion and sauté over medium heat until the garlic turns golden brown. Add the sweet potatoes and stock. Bring to a boil. Then turn the heat down and simmer for 10 minutes, until the sweet potatoes are soft. Wash the watercress well. Save a handful of leaves to be used as a garnish later. Add the rest of the watercress and the milk to the sweet potatoes and simmer for about 10 minutes. Remove from heat. Purée in batches in the blender, and then return to the pot. Heat until the first bubbles appear around the edge, then stir in the egg substitute until the soup thickens.

Note: This soup can be reheated if not allowed to boil. You may use homemade stock as long as it has not been made with vegetables that have high sodium content. You might use low-sodium vegetable powder to be sure.

CREAMY TOMATO SOUP

1 butternut squash (½ cup pulp)
½ tomato (¼ cup juice)
½ cup plus 3 T plain soy yogurt
½ cup chopped tomatoes
2 tsp chopped fresh dill
½ tsp sea salt

¼ tsp pepper
2 T plain yogurt (for garnish)
2 T soy Parmesan cheese (for garnish)
2 sprigs fresh dill (for garnish)

Separately juice the squash and tomato to get ½ cup of squash pulp and ¼ cup of tomato juice. In a medium-size saucepan, combine the pulp, juice, and soy yogurt. Bring to a simmer over medium-low heat and cook uncovered for 10–15 minutes. Add the chopped tomato, 2 tsp dill, salt, and pepper, and remove from the heat. Serve hot or cold, garnished with the yogurt, Parmesan cheese, and dill sprigs, if desired.

PAPAYA NECTAR SOUP

4 small papayas, peeled, seeded, and cut into 2-inch pieces (about 8 cups)
16 large nectarines, pitted and quartered
4 large limes, peeled
⅓ cup lemon-flavored nondairy yogurt
fresh mint to garnish

Separately juice papayas, nectarines, and limes. Serve chilled in bowls garnished with a dollop of yogurt and mint leaves.

Breakfast Dishes
TIPS
- Grains cooked in advance may be reheated by steaming.
- Grains are more flavorful when cooked with ½ teaspoon sea salt per cup of dry grain.
- Although unhulled barley is most desirable because it is the whole grain, it has a longer cooking time than "pearled" barley; look for the darker varieties of pearled barley found in health food stores, as they are minimally processed.
- Grade B or C maple syrup is less processed than Grade A, retaining more of its natural minerals.

BLUEBERRY BREAKFAST TREAT

1 cup brown rice, cooked (room temperature)
½ cup blueberries, cut in half
2 T sunflower seeds
sprinkle of unsweetened, flaked coconut

Combine all ingredients and mix well.

BLUEBERRY-BANANA PANCAKES

½ cup spelt flour
½ cup wheat germ
1 tsp baking powder
1 tsp baking soda
dash of ground nutmeg
1 cup plain soy yogurt
½ cup thinly sliced bananas
¾ cup fresh or frozen blueberries
¼ cup oil (sunflower, soy, or safflower oil)

In a medium-size mixing bowl, combine the flour, wheat germ, baking powder, baking soda, and nutmeg. Mix well with a fork to remove lumps. Mix in the yogurt, bananas, and blueberries. Heat the oil in a large skillet over medium heat. Pour 3–4 tablespoons of batter into the oil at a time and cook for 2–3 minutes on each side until light brown.

BLUEBERRY BUCKWHEAT-SOY-BANANA PANCAKES

2 T egg substitute
2 T vanilla extract
1 banana, mashed
½ cup rice milk
½ cup spelt flour
½ cup buckwheat flour
½ cup soy flour

1 tsp baking powder
1 tsp baking soda
4 T raisins
½ cup blueberries
4 T canola oil
3 T shredded unsweetened coconut
   (optional)

In a medium-size mixing bowl, combine the egg substitute, vanilla, banana, and milk, mixing with a fork until well blended. In a separate bowl, combine the flours, baking powder, and baking soda, mixing well. Add the flour mixture to the banana and milk mixture, blending well with a spoon. Stir in the raisins and blueberries. Heat the oil in a large skillet over medium heat. Pour in 2–3 tablespoons of batter at a time and cook for 3–5 minutes on each side until light brown. Garnish with coconut.

CREAM OF BARLEY

½ cup silken tofu
2 T chopped walnuts
1 banana, mashed

1 T pure maple syrup
½ cup cooked pearled barley
2 T protein powder

In a saucepan, combine all of the ingredients except barley and protein powder over low heat, until creamy. Add barley, stirring until hot. Sprinkle protein powder on top and serve immediately.

NUTTY BANANA BREAKFAST

6 ounces barley, cooked
3 ounces banana, mashed

1½ ounces walnuts, chopped
2 T agave sweetener

Combine all ingredients and mix well.

NUTTY OATMEAL

6 ounces oatmeal, cooked (room
   temperature)
3 ounces pears, cut into bite-size
   pieces

1½ ounces pecans, chopped
1 T honey

Combine all ingredients. Mix well.

RICE AND STRAWBERRIES

1 cup rice milk
⅛ to ½ tsp pure vanilla extract
1 T pure maple syrup
½ cup raw cashews

1 pinch sea salt
½ cup sliced strawberries
1 cup cooked brown rice, hot

In a blender, combine rice milk, vanilla extract, maple syrup, cashews, and salt. Sprinkle strawberries over hot rice. Pour the cashew sauce over all. Serve immediately.

Main Dishes

BRAZILIAN RICE

2 T sunflower oil
3 ounces cauliflower florets, in bite-size pieces
2 T fresh chopped parsley
½ tsp soy sauce
½ tsp salt
3 ounces black beans, cooked
3 ounces brown rice, cooked
3 ounces avocado, sliced

Preheat the oven to 350°F. Lightly grease a 4-×-8 baking pan with sunflower oil. Steam the cauliflower about 5 minutes. Combine all the ingredients except for the avocado. Mix well. Transfer to baking pan and bake for 15 minutes. Garnish with avocado slices.

CHICKPEA HUMMUS WITH TOASTED PITA TRIANGLES

1 sweet onion, chopped
2 cloves garlic, minced
1 can garbanzo beans or
  chickpeas, drained
½ cup tahini (sesame butter)
½ cup lemon juice
½ tsp pepper
⅛ tsp cayenne pepper
⅓ cup chopped fresh parsley
  (optional)
½ cup water
pita bread
3 T olive oil
garlic powder or garlic salt, to taste

Sauté onion and garlic in oil until onion is transparent. Put into blender or food processor with garbanzo beans or chickpeas, tahini, lemon juice, pepper, cayenne pepper, and parsley. Blend until smooth, adding a little water if necessary to achieve desired consistency. Cut pita bread into triangles, paint lightly with olive oil, and sprinkle with garlic powder or garlic salt. Broil until lightly browned.

GARY'S VEGETABLE PAN

2 tomatoes (½ cup juice)
1 pound extra-firm tofu, cut into 1-inch cubes
2 T canola oil
½ cup yellow onions, chopped
2 cups frozen peas
1 cup tomatoes, chopped
½ cup plain soy milk
3 tsp apple cider vinegar
½ cup arugula, finely chopped
2 green chili peppers, finely chopped
3 cloves garlic, crushed
2 tsp ginger root, grated
1 tsp ground coriander
1 tsp ground turmeric
½ tsp chili powder
1½ tsp sea salt

Juice tomatoes to get ½ cup of juice. In a large frying pan, brown tofu in oil over high heat. Add onions. Sauté for 2–3 minutes, or until onions are soft. Reduce heat to medium-low. Add the ½ cup of tomato juice, peas, chopped tomatoes, soy milk, cider vinegar, arugula, chili peppers, garlic, ginger, coriander, turmeric, chili powder, and sea salt. Simmer, uncovered, for 5 minutes. Serve with fresh green salad.

GARY'S VEGGIEBALL STEW

1 tsp sea salt
⅛ tsp white pepper
1 tsp Worcestershire sauce
1 tsp grated lemon peel
½ tsp dried thyme
1 T curry powder
1 tsp tamari sauce
1 stalk celery, chopped
1 scallion, chopped
2 T egg substitute
1 T Bragg Liquid Aminos
4 ounces seitan, chopped
½ cup spelt flour
1 T extra-virgin olive oil
4 cups filtered water
1 cup yellow squash, sliced
1 small turnip, boiled and cubed
1 medium red potato, boiled and shredded
1 cup fresh tomato, peeled, cored, and chopped
1 leek with top sliced off
vegetable broth bouillon cubes, enough for 1 quart
1 T chopped fresh dill

In a medium-size bowl, combine salt, pepper, Worcestershire sauce, lemon peel, thyme, curry, tamari, celery, scallion, egg substitute, Bragg Aminos, and chopped seitan. Shape into 1-inch balls and roll in spelt flour. Heat oil in a skillet and brown the balls, turning gently between a fork and a spoon. Set aside. Save and set aside drippings. In a large saucepan, with 4 cups water, place squash, turnip, potato, tomato, leek, and vegetable bouillon cubes. Boil on medium heat for approximately 30 minutes. Add veggieballs to soup and heat for 5–7 minutes. Sprinkle dill on top.

GOOD SHEPHERD'S PIE

1 large baking potato, peeled and diced
2 T sunflower seed oil
½ cup rice milk
1 T curry powder
½ tsp celery salt
⅛ T freshly ground black pepper
1 T olive oil
1 clove garlic, minced
1 medium onion, chopped
1 scallion, chopped
½ pound vegetarian meat substitute (texturized vegetable protein, TVP)
1 vegetable bouillon cube
3 ounces tomato paste
½ cup anchovy paste
⅛ tsp sage
1 T spelt flour
1 tsp parsley flakes
1 tsp dried tarragon
½ cup white wine
½ can adzuki beans, cooked
1 pinch paprika

Cook potato in boiling, salted water. Drain and mash, and add the sunflower seed oil and rice milk. Season with curry powder, celery salt, and pepper. Heat olive oil and sauté garlic, onion, and scallion until soft. Add the meat substitute and stir until brown and flavors are married, about 5 minutes. Crumble the vegetable bouillon and stir it into the onion mixture. Stir in tomato paste, anchovy paste, sage, flour, parsley, and tarragon. Add the wine and continue stirring for a few minutes. Cover and simmer on low for 10 additional minutes. Preheat oven to 350°F. Lightly coat soufflé dish or bread pan with oil. Spread onion mixture on bottom of the dish. Follow with a layer of cooked adzuki beans and then mashed potatoes, and sprinkle with paprika. Bake for 30 minutes, then brown under broiler for 1 minute and serve.

INDONESIAN KALE

1 cup onions, chopped
3 cups fresh tomatoes, chopped
½ cup extra-virgin olive oil
4 cups fresh or frozen kale, chopped
4 cups diced red potatoes, steamed 15 minutes
4 cloves garlic, sliced
2–3 T curry powder, dissolved in 2 T water
½ tsp ground allspice
½ tsp ground ginger
½ tsp paprika
2 T salt

In a large saucepan, sauté the onions and tomatoes in oil over medium heat for 15 minutes. Add remaining ingredients and cook additional 5 minutes.

ITALIAN VEGETABLE STEW

2 T olive oil
1 large onion, sliced thin
3 cloves garlic, pressed
1 red pepper, coarsely chopped
1 green pepper, coarsely chopped
2 carrots, sliced thin
2 small zucchini, sliced
½ bunch broccoli, cut into stalks
½ head cauliflower, cut into florets

2 tomatoes, chopped
2 cups red wine
1 T honey
1 T basil
1 tsp oregano
2 tsp parsley flakes
1 tsp tamari (soy sauce)
1 cup grated soy Parmesan cheese

Heat the oil in a large skillet and add the onion, garlic, red pepper, green pepper, and carrots. Sauté for 5 minutes. Add the zucchini and sauté for 5 minutes longer. Stir in the broccoli, cauliflower, tomatoes, wine, honey, basil, oregano, parsley, and tamari. Cover and simmer for 25 minutes, stirring occasionally. Place in an oiled casserole, top with soy Parmesan cheese, and bake for 20 minutes at 350°F.

MACARONI MARCONI

½ pound quinoa pasta
10 artichoke hearts
½ pound salmon fillets, cubed
½ tsp sea salt
½ tsp cayenne
½ lemon
3 cloves garlic, minced
2 ounces sun-dried tomatoes
2 T extra-virgin olive oil
1 sprig fresh basil, chopped
15 green olives, pitted and sliced
½ cup grated soy or rice Parmesan, optional

Cook pasta. Steam artichoke hearts until tender. Season salmon with salt, cayenne, and lemon. In a skillet, sauté garlic with sun-dried tomatoes in the olive oil, 3 minutes. Add salmon, basil, and olives, and cook until the salmon flakes when tested with a fork, about 5 minutes more. In a large bowl, toss salmon mixture with the pasta and Parmesan, and serve.

ORIGINAL BROCCOLI STIR-FRY

1 cup firm tofu
2 cups broccoli florets
2 T hot sesame oil
2 T tamari sauce
½ tsp cayenne pepper
1 tsp grated fresh ginger
3 cloves garlic, minced

In a medium-size saucepan, sauté tofu and broccoli in oil for 3 minutes over medium heat. Remove from pan and place mixture in a bowl. Combine remaining ingredients in the saucepan. Cook over medium heat until mixture simmers, 1 minute. Add broccoli mixture and cook, covered, for 2 minutes. Stir well. Serve with short-grain brown rice or Far East rice noodles.

PASTA FAGIOLI (BEAN SOUP)

3 cloves garlic, diced
½ onion, diced
2 T olive oil
two 28-ounce cans of tomato
  purée
½ tsp garlic powder

½ tsp oregano
salt and pepper to taste
1 can cannellini beans or white
  kidney beans
3 cups Ditallini pasta or other
  small noodle, cooked

Sauté garlic and onion in olive oil. Add tomato purée, bring to a boil, and add spices and beans. Cook for ½ hour over low to medium heat. Add cooked pasta; if too thick, add water to reach desired consistency.

POTATO CHOWDER

1 pound golden potatoes, peeled
  and cut into ½-inch cubes
½ pound purple potatoes, peeled
  and cut into 1-inch cubes
2 T extra-virgin olive oil
1 medium onion, chopped
2 stalks celery, minced
4 cloves garlic, minced
1 yellow bell pepper, diced
2 scallions, white only, chopped
1 T sherry (optional)
3 cups filtered water
1 cup plain soy milk
½ cup diced carrots

1 bay leaf
1 small jalapeño pepper
1 tsp freshly ground black pepper
1 tsp sea salt
1 tsp dried thyme seeds
1 tsp ground sage
1 tsp dried basil
1 tsp Pick a Pepper or Tabasco
  Sauce
1 T mustard seeds
1 T fennel seeds
1 T honey
parsley and Hungarian paprika
  (for garnish)

Steam potatoes for 10 minutes. In a stockpot, heat oil over medium heat and sauté onion, celery, garlic, yellow pepper, scallions, and sherry (optional). Add water, soy milk, carrots, and steamed potatoes to the sautéed vegetables. Add bay leaf, jalapeño, pepper, salt, thyme, sage, basil, pepper sauce, mustard seeds, fennel seeds, and honey. Stir and simmer an additional 15 minutes. Garnish with parsley and Hungarian paprika.

RATATOUILLE

4 T plus ¼ cup extra-virgin olive oil
1 small eggplant, peeled and cubed
1 small yellow squash, cubed
½ cup shallots, minced
1 scallion, chopped
2 cloves garlic, pressed
1 small zucchini, cubed
¼ tsp thyme
¼ tsp dried basil
1 small onion, chopped
2 T dulse leaves, minced
½ stalk celery, chopped
⅓ cup sun-dried tomatoes, reconstituted in ⅓ cup water
1 T curry powder
sea salt
freshly ground black pepper
½ cup raw sunflower seeds

Heat olive oil in a large skillet over medium heat. Add eggplant, yellow squash, shallots, scallion, garlic, and zucchini. Cook, stirring, 3 minutes. Add thyme, basil, onion, dulse, and celery, and cook another 3 minutes. Add sun-dried tomatoes, curry powder, and sea salt and fresh pepper to taste. Sprinkle with sunflower seeds and serve warm.

SWEET KIDNEY BEAN MASH

1 pound sweet potatoes or yams, scrubbed well and cut into 2-inch-thick
  slices (about 2 cups)
½ cup extra-virgin olive oil
one 8-ounce yellow onion, peeled and finely chopped
2 large celery stalks, finely chopped
3 large cloves garlic, peeled and coarsely chopped
1 pound cooked kidney beans, rinsed and drained
½ cup freshly squeezed lime juice
10 large basil leaves
1 tsp sea salt
1 tsp ground cumin
1 tsp ground chili powder
freshly ground black pepper to taste (optional)
8 slices whole grain country bread or millet bread, cut ½ inch thick

Place the sweet potato slices in a steamer set into a large pot containing 1 inch of water. Cook, covered, over moderate to high heat until the potatoes are tender when a fork is inserted into their centers, about 15–20 minutes. Remove the steamer and run the potatoes under cool water until they can be handled comfortably. Using a small paring knife, remove and discard the peels.

In a medium saucepan, combine the oil, onion, celery, and garlic. Sauté over moderate heat for 5–7 minutes, or until the onions are translucent. In a food processor, using a metal blade, combine the sautéed vegetables with the sweet potatoes, beans, lime juice, basil leaves, salt, cumin, chili powder, and black pepper. Process together until smooth and creamy, about 2 minutes. Set aside.

Lightly toast the bread on both sides. Spread bread slices with sweet mash and serve warm.

TANTALIZING TEMPEH DINNER

2 T soy oil
½ ounce dulse, dry
3 ounces chickpeas, cooked
3 ounces soybean sprouts
3 ounces broccoli florets, in bite-size pieces
3 ounces tempeh, cut into ½-inch cubes
1 tsp fresh chives, chopped
1 tsp onion, minced
½ tsp salt

Preheat oven to 350°F. Lightly grease a 4-×-8 baking pan with soy oil. Soak and rinse dulse 2 or 3 times in cold water. Combine with chickpeas, soybean sprouts, broccoli, tempeh, chives, onion, and salt, and mix well. Transfer to baking pan and bake for 20 minutes.

TEX-MEX TOFU SCRAMBLER

½ cup sunflower seeds
6 T extra-virgin olive oil
four 1-ounce slices Fakin' Bacon
    (tempeh, available in health
    food stores)
½ cup lecithin granules (optional)
1 T onion powder
1 T dry mustard
1 T dried basil
1 T ground turmeric
1 T ground cumin
1 T celery salt
1 T sea salt
1 pound soft tofu, well drained
    and crumbled
1 cup mushrooms, sliced
3 T tamari soy sauce
one 6-ounce Vidalia onion, peeled
    and finely chopped
4 large cloves garlic, peeled and
    finely chopped
one 8-ounce yellow bell pepper,
    cored, seeded, and finely
    chopped
½ cup zucchini, finely chopped
one 6-ounce tomato, cored and
    finely chopped
1 ripe Haas avocado, peeled,
    halved, pitted, and finely
    chopped
1 T balsamic vinegar
½ cup fresh cilantro, finely
    chopped
freshly ground black pepper
    to taste (for garnish)
2 large limes, sliced into
    1-inch-thick wedges
    (for garnish)

In a large cast-iron frying pan, over moderate to low heat, roast the sunflower seeds until golden and transfer to a small dish. Set aside. Preheat the broiler and brush the frying pan with 2 tablespoons oil. Evenly space the tempeh in the pan and broil for 5 minutes, or until golden. Remove the pan from the oven, transfer the "bacon" to a paper-towel-lined plate, and set aside. In a small mixing bowl, combine the lecithin, onion powder, mustard, basil, turmeric, cumin, celery salt, and sea salt. Stir together until well combined and set aside. In a large mixing bowl, toss together 2 tablespoons of the oil with the tofu and the spice mixture until well combined. Set aside. In the frying pan, combine the remaining 2 tablespoons oil with the mushrooms and tamari. Toss together until well mixed and broil for 5 minutes, or until the mushrooms are golden. Remove the pan from the oven and toss in the prepared tofu, onion, garlic, yellow pepper, zucchini, tomato, avocado, vinegar, cilantro, and black pepper until well combined. Return to the broiler and broil, mixing occasionally, until golden, about 10 minutes. Serve hot, garnished with "bacon," sunflower seeds, and lime, accompanied by whole grain toast.

Desserts

BLACKBERRY NECTARINE FRUIT SALAD

1 large cantaloupe, peeled, seeded, and cut into 1-inch pieces (about 4 cups)
8 large nectarines, pitted and sliced (about 4 cups)
4 cups blackberries
1 T freshly squeezed lemon juice
3 T freshly squeezed lime juice
2 T powdered brown rice syrup (optional)

In a large bowl, combine the cantaloupe, nectarines, and blackberries. Drizzle the juices onto the fruit and gently toss together until well coated. Spoon into small bowls, sprinkle on the powder, and serve.

CAROB POWER BROWNIES

½ cup sunflower seeds
1½ cups brown rice flour
½ cup carob powder
½ T baking powder
½ T ground nutmeg
½ T sea salt
½ cup extra-virgin olive oil
5 large bananas, peeled and coarsely chopped (about 2½ cups)
1 cup apple juice
1 cup apricot juice
1 T honey
1½ tsp pure banana flavor
1 cup walnuts, coarsely chopped
1 cup oat bran
½ cup plus 2 T rice bran
½ cup dairy-free carob chips

Preheat oven to 350°F. Line two 12-well muffin tins with paper baking cups and set aside. Using a mini food processor or coffee grinder, process the sunflower seeds until powder-fine. Transfer to a mixing bowl and set aside. To make the brownies, in a large mixing bowl, sift together the flour, carob powder, baking powder, nutmeg, and salt. Whisk together until well mixed. Set aside. In a food processor, using the metal blade, combine the oil and bananas. Process until creamy, about 1 minute. Pour in the apple juice, apricot juice, honey, and banana flavor. Process until well blended. With a rubber spatula, gradually add the wet ingredients to the dry, making sure they are well blended before each addition. Scrape off any excess batter from the side of the bowl. Stir in the walnuts, oat bran, rice bran, and chips until well mixed. Spoon the batter into the prepared muffin tins (the wells will be half full). Bake in the middle level of the preheated oven for 35–40 minutes. For uniformity in baking, rotate the tin from front to back halfway through the baking period. The brownies are done when a tester inserted in the center comes out clean. Remove the brownies from the oven and let cool completely, about 15–20 minutes. Serve with a glass of rice milk, soy milk, or nut milk.

CHERRY GRAPE KANTEN

6 cups pineapple juice
½ cup plus 2 T agar flakes (available at your local health food store)
8 medium ripe peaches, peeled, pitted, and sliced (about 3 cups)
½ large pineapple, peeled, cored, and cut into 1-inch pieces (about 2 cups)
2 cups seedless green grapes
two 12-ounce packages frozen pitted cherries
2 T freshly squeezed lemon juice

In a medium-size saucepan, bring the pineapple juice to a boil over high heat. Reduce heat to moderate and stir in the agar. Simmer uncovered, stirring occasionally, for 10 minutes, or until the agar is completely dissolved. In a large mixing bowl, toss the peaches, pineapple, grapes, and cherries together with the lemon juice until well combined. Transfer to a 7-×-11-inch baking dish and pour in the pineapple juice mixture. Let cool for 15 minutes; then refrigerate for 30–45 minutes, or until congealed. Spoon into small bowls and serve.

COLD CHERRY SOUP

2 cups of cherries, pitted and stemmed
1 lemon, peeled and quartered
1 cup strawberries, hulled
1 cup blueberries
½ cup agar
cinnamon, to taste
1 orange, peeled and in wedges

Juice the cherries and lemon. In a blender, blend cherry juice together with the strawberries, blueberries, and agar. Serve in a bowl with cinnamon garnish and orange wedges.

HEAVENLY ROASTED NUTS

1 cup walnuts
1 T honey
1 tsp extra-virgin olive oil
1 tsp freshly squeezed lemon juice

Preheat oven to 350°F. Line an 11-×-15-inch cookie sheet with parchment paper and set aside. In a medium-size mixing bowl, toss together the nuts, honey, oil, and lemon juice until well combined. Evenly spread the nuts on the prepared sheet. Bake on the middle rack of the preheated oven for 8–10 minutes, or until the nuts are golden. Remove sheet from the oven and slide the parchment paper to a wire rack until the nuts are completely cool (about 10 minutes). Serve alone or use these as a topping for cereal, salads, nondairy yogurt, or nondairy frozen dessert.

PART III

APPENDICES

PURCHASING VITAMINS, SUPPLEMENTS, AND HERBAL REMEDIES

When I am talking with people in my travels, one of the questions they most frequently ask me is "How can I be sure I am choosing a high-quality supplement?" With the rise in popularity of nutritional supplements, it can be confusing to know how to purchase high-quality vitamins, minerals, and supplements.

Natural health stores or groceries stock most of the vitamins, supplements, and herbs that I recommend in this book. Even some mainstream grocery stores carry many of the vitamins and supplements mentioned in this book. If you are able to use the Internet, it is easy to research and purchase supplements and herbal remedies online.

VITAMINS AND SUPPLEMENTS

When shopping for vitamins and supplements, there are a few important questions you should ask:

- How does the manufacturer select their ingredients?
- What is the specific formula of the vitamin or supplement?
- What is the potency level of the vitamin or supplement?
- Does the manufacturer test for quality control, and if so, how?
- Are the vitamins natural (that is, from food sources) or are there added ingredients?

You may wonder whether it is better to choose tablets, capsules, powders, or liquids when purchasing vitamins and supplements. Generally speaking, tablets have a long shelf life, but can contain fillers and stabilizers that may cause allergic reactions. Capsules are generally used for fat-soluble and powdered supplements. The powdered type is most rapidly absorbed and generally contains no additives. The liquid forms may contain coloring agents or sweeteners.

Multivitamins may be useful in combining vitamins and minerals that are more effective when taken together (such as a B-complex vitamin). Most multivitamins combine vitamins and minerals in complementary doses. In some of the protocols, I recommend doses higher than those found in multivitamins. For that reason, with the exception of a B-complex vitamin, I recommend buying vitamins and supplements individually.

Finally, when purchasing supplements, remember these important points:

- Buy from organic sources whenever possible.
- Avoid artificial ingredients.
- If you have food sensitivities, buy hypoallergenic products. Avoid wheat, yeast, and corn.
- Always examine the expiration date before purchasing.
- If you have any questions or doubts about a product, never hesitate to contact the manufacturer and ask them questions. A reputable company will not hesitate to address concerns.

For a more detailed discussion of vitamins and supplements, go to www.garynull.com.

HERBAL REMEDIES

If you are taking herbs, it is essential to take them in proper dosages, for they contain powerful ingredients. For centuries, people have been taking herbs to treat various conditions. When taken in the correct manner, herbs do not have the side effects that traditional medicines may cause. If herbs are used randomly or indiscriminately, however, they may produce unwanted side effects. If you are taking prescription or over-the-counter medications, you should talk with your health care provider before taking any herbal remedies, as some may have adverse interactions with medications.

Herbs may be taken in their natural forms of leaves, barks, or roots by brewing them in teas. More commonly, herbs are taken in capsules or tinctures. Herbs can be used in compresses, applied externally with essential oils, or infused in teas, ointments, or salves.

For more information on herbal remedies, including hundreds of scientific studies on the efficacy of herbs for impacting various conditions, along with recommended dosages, go to www.garynull.com.

TESTIMONIALS

Depression

I was dissatisfied with my body. My energy was low, and I was very overweight. My acquaintances and friends were depressing me to the point of irritability. I had a fear of public speaking and did not know where to turn for guidance. I joined Gary's health support group. I lost sixteen pounds without dieting. My increasing energy made me feel young again. I need less sleep and find I am not distracted with other people's petty, unimportant issues. My toxic relationships were dismissed. My self-esteem replaced them. I learned to be the real me, healthy and vital.

—Alexandra M.

Mental Fatigue

I was concerned about my health. My blood pressure and cholesterol were elevated. I had a stressful life due to being mentally fatigued and could not control these feelings. I suffered an acid reflux condition that I assumed was being caused by my job. My body was falling apart. I detoxed and carefully followed Gary's protocol. I felt stronger each week and released stress each day. My blood pressure is now normal, my digestion is improved, and I lost fifteen pounds. I do aerobics at home in the morning, yoga during evening hours, bike, walk, and run. My uncluttered environment and journal writing give me a new constructive outlet.

—Alice

Brain Allergies

I had many allergies and frequent upper-respiratory infections. My life was unmanageable and my stress was overwhelming. My blood pressure and cholesterol were elevated. I heard about Gary Null's support groups and detoxification. I needed to change and decided to enter a group as soon as one was formed. That was the beginning of the best part of my life. My energy built, my headaches stopped, and my cholesterol and blood pressure lowered. I have a new body since exercising, using weights, doing chi gong, and deep breathing. I feel calm, more patient, and less irritable. I love my food and progressive life.

—Bob

Depression

I weighed 210 pounds, smoked three packs of cigarettes a day, drank alcohol, felt depressed, had knee pains and upper-respiratory infections. One day I looked at the very aged man in the mirror and was shocked. Today I follow Gary Null's protocol. I drink purified water, use supplements and feel terrific. I haven't had a cold in five years, no more upper-respiratory infections. I follow an organic, vegan diet and do not take vaccines. My neighbors tell me I look forty-five years old. They admire my changes. I appreciate my healthy lifestyle. I am confident and pleased with my life and I am no longer depressed.

—Job

Brain Trauma

In 1989 I attended a Gary Null retreat. I learned the benefits of vegetarianism, juicing, supplements, and meditation. In 1994 I became disabled because of carbon monoxide poisoning. I am still in the process of recovery. I no longer work. I cannot see computer screens. Surgery for two detached retinas affected my eyesight. My blood pressure was extremely high. My heartbeat accelerated to a dangerous level. I took several pharmaceutical drugs to control these conditions. A few years later seizures began with Alzheimer's-like symptoms. Abnormally severe edema in my legs incapacitated me. I was in a coma for sixty days. Nursing home care was considered. My health took an upward turn on the Gary Null protocol. Juicing, stress management, and homework opened me to my potentials and purpose in life. I discovered the best of what works and realized I was not doing anything worthwhile. Today I no longer need a compressor for leg edema. My leg size decreased 30 percent. I sleep less, lost twenty-three pounds, and exercise with hand weights. I recently received a

Bowflex to build my upper body. My blood pressure is lower. My brain speed seems to be faster.

—Michael

Migraine

I was labeled disabled for four years. Migraine headaches caused me to be bedridden, and I used pain medication for a spinal disk injury. I was swollen after eating my usual meat, wheat, sugar, coffee, and dairy. My cholesterol was high. Candida plagued my body. I threw up after meals and was stressed by anxiety attacks. One day after reading one of Gary's books I saw him on PBS. I joined a support group in 1994. I attended classes open to change, and after two weeks on the protocol being vegan, organic, and never returning to toxic foods, the change began. I exercise in a rehab center for my back problem. Probiotics and sensible eating eliminated throwing up. I am a vegetarian cook and intend to study vegetarian meal preparation. Back pain is sporadic and not as acute. I am still in recovery but use no medication. I never looked at life as I do now.

—Barbara

Memory Loss

I was bedridden for two weeks with Epstein-Barr disease and could not walk more than three minutes at a time. I lost some of my memory. I returned to work but only put in five hours a day, and went to bed as soon as I returned home. Stair climbing was difficult. My physician could do no more and suggested I do independent research. A homeopathic examination revealed food sensitivities. The day I watched Gary on PBS changed my life. I donated to the station and soon joined a support group. Today I carefully follow the protocol. I gave up chocolate without difficulty. At first the new food choices were difficult to accept, but today I am vegan and feel 1,000 percent better. I work seven hours a day and exercise after work. I walk one and a half hours and am training to race-walk in the New York Marathon. I still need eight hours of sleep, possibly because of Epstein-Barr, but my waking hours are productive. With a clear mind, good memory, energy and concentration I plan future occupations in art and volunteer work.

—Cathy T.

Insomnia

I could not sleep well and was tired all day long. I wanted to be healthy and change my work. I decided to join a support group. I heard members of Gary's groups speak of their successes. I intended to change my work and life. I was overweight. My hair and nails were weak. I had a swollen knee because of three automobile accidents. I suffered with skin eruptions. The group had a wonderful effect. I became friends with several people and spoke to them during the week. We motivated each other. Today I am twenty-five pounds thinner. My hair and nails grow rapidly. The swelling in my knee has lessened. I no longer have skin eruptions. My energy is high all day long because I sleep well. I have also actualized a new career.

—Eileen

Anxiety

I used to feel no one understood my problem and fear of isolation. I was reticent about meeting with a group of people to improve my life, but I did and felt that the group enhanced my progress. I stayed on the protocol and lost ten pounds. I now feel joy, happiness—I feel really good about myself. I can now easily help other people. Praying and listening to my inner voice brought good results. The protocol cleaned my body and mind.

—Kenneth L.

Brain Trauma

Brain surgery left me with numb fingers and cold extremities. I had flulike symptoms, a constant "frog" in my throat, fatigue in the morning, tinnitus, dizziness, constipation, and a general lack of motivation that interfered with my work performance. I was angry and soon went on disability. The first time Gary Null spoke about support groups on his show I listened but did nothing. At that stage I could not really help myself. Feeling totally locked in, I pulled up some inner courage and went to the first meeting. I began the protocol. In a short amount of time it was evident the protocol was working. I began to feel better, the pains and other symptoms lessened. As I continued and listened to the lectures, which were quite penetrating and motivating, I noticed all the symptoms I once had were gone. Today I am a functioning, healthy woman.

—Yvonne

Depression

I was prescribed Prozac for Multi-Menopausal Syndrome by my gynecologist. I gained weight and lost energy. My hair and nails were weak. I had difficulty sleeping and felt depressed. I thought I followed a sensible eating plan. I did not *connect food and aging. I began the detox protocol carefully and followed it diligently. I wanted to reverse my aging and clean my system out. I lost weight and am keeping it off. I have good energy. My hair and nails are growing to pre-menopausal thickness and strength. I discontinued the Prozac when I began the protocol and am not depressed. I sleep well, look well, and get healthier each day.*

—Maria R.

Memory Loss

At age seventy-five, we were not happy with symptoms of getting old. We both had memory difficulties. I did not like to be a homebody and wanted this part of our lives to be active. There is so much to experience and learn. We joined a support group and feel we have reversed aging. We follow the protocol and noticed we have increased brain power. It is sad watching our friends fail physically. They are closed to the ideas of detoxification and diet changes. We are the only couple in our group not taking medications. I study piano and am writing a book. This is a wonderful time of life.

—Wilma and Myron

Headaches

My blood pressure was a bit high and I did get headaches. I was curious about this thing called a detox protocol. I did not feel unhealthy, but I decided to attend a group and see if it impacts in any way. I came to each meeting and listened and learned. I lost weight without dieting. My waistline is smaller. My blood pressure is normal. I need less sleep and my headaches are gone. The protocol and the science behind it are valid. It was a wonderful experience.

—Bob

Depression

I was depressed and overweight, uncomfortable with the extra pounds. I held anger in and did not discuss, understand, or share my feelings with anyone. I was afraid to take risks, such as asking for a raise. Being timid and angry was not a good place to be. I knew and trusted Gary Null, so I joined a group to see if I could be happy and make changes. I am on the protocol and love it. My depression lifted as my health increased. I exercise without fear of injury. I lost twenty pounds and my energy is high. I cope, do not hold anger in, and speak my mind. I spoke up at work and got a raise.

—Maria T.

Memory Loss

My memory has significantly improved. I can now connect the names and faces of my friends. I am calmer and more relaxed. My energy level has gone up. I can get through the day without feeling drowsy.

—Joyce C.

Depression/Anxiety

I am much more relaxed, am more able to handle stress, and I need less sleep. My vision is clearer, my hair has gone back to its original color, and I feel twenty years younger. My meditation is now much deeper and richer and I have less anger and depression. I feel sexy (at fifty-nine!) and I'm thinking about companionship. People who haven't seen me blurt out, "My God, what have you done to yourself? You look fabulous!" I lost sixteen pounds, went down two sizes in clothing, and my abdomen went from forty-four inches to thirty-nine inches. Most days I do twenty to thirty stretching exercises, and I am now willing to challenge my values and beliefs.

—Molly

Headaches

I feel energetic, attractive, and strong. The changes I was able to make during this protocol were more marked than any changes I have been able to make in several years. I followed the protocol closely and I no longer get headaches, whereas before I usually got at least one severe headache a month. I lost twelve pounds and several inches from my hips and waist. My blood pressure dropped to 102/60. My self-confidence and energy level rose to a new high. I received many comments on my shiny hair, and people commented on how nice my skin was. I feel more confident, positive, and clearheaded, and able to focus on other life goals. I feel like a different person—stronger, happier, and enthusiastic.

—Elaine

Depression

Mentally, I am more clear-thinking, making decisions regarding my life and business quicker, as opposed to laboring over them. I have no depression, but a general feeling of grounding and balance. Affirmations work.

—Liz

Headaches

I am migraine-free. My circulation has improved in my fingers and toes and I have lots of energy. My sleep has improved and I wake up energized.

—Jayne

Memory Loss

I had heard about Gary Null from a friend, who had been listening to his daily radio program in New York. I decided to go to his office, where he had mentioned there would be a support group. I was showing signs of Alzheimer's that were getting worse and worse. I was overweight, and I had blotches of skin discoloration all over my body. I thought Gary's protocol was too harsh to try, so I decided not to go on it. After a few months, however, when my condition got worse, I went back to his office and immediately began the program.

I had not exercised for quite some time. Now, every day, I would set aside time to walk. My bowel habits became more regular, and suddenly I was remembering things that I used to forget. I could easily recall the names of friends I would run into on the street, where before I would have difficulty doing so. I feel that Gary's protocol has given me my life back, for it doesn't matter how good of shape your body is in if your mind is forgetful.

—Rita

Depression

I feel a balance, peacefulness, quietness, and contentment. My depression is gone. This is new for me, I feel joyful. I am now walking two to three miles four or five times per week. I feel lighter, see the world in a more positive way, and feel content and happier. People are telling me how great I look.

—Louise

Memory Loss

I am now in my early forties and I feel great! I feel better than I did in my twenties. I am generally sharper, with better memory, and I am experiencing greater mental stability. I have much greater focus and discipline about my daily life and my long-term life goals. I exercise, meditate, eat right, and take supplements daily. Dry skin on my feet cleared up, thinning hair improved, allergies are gone. I have not had any colds or flu since beginning the program. I need less sleep and wake up refreshed and ready for a wonderful day. The dietary changes expanded my food choices. In place of meat, dairy, sugar, and wheat items, I found a whole new world of grains, beans, legumes, fruits, vegetables, and fish to eat. I enjoy exercising but never made time for it on a regular basis, and now I do. In summary, I have achieved that which I set out to do: I am healthier in body, mind, and spirit. I look forward to waking up each day with good health, happiness, and fulfillment.

—Pat

Depression

I feel more worthy of living and of being alive. At the start of the program I didn't care! My depression has diminished noticeably. Life is no longer happening to me. I am involved. I'm not as timid and I cry less. I am more in control of my emotions. I am happier.

—Jennie

Brain Allergies

As a child my food sensitivities were treated with antibiotics and medications to no avail. I was weak in every aspect of my being, and pale with dark circles under my eyes. Within two weeks on Gary Null's allergy protocol, I felt remarkably better. Nine months later I find I can tolerate most all foods. My thinking is clear, moodiness, depression, lethargy, and poor complexion have reversed. I feel vital, healthy, and alive. I anticipate studying Oriental Medicine and continue research on internal energy.

—Peter

Brain Trauma

In February 1997 I had brain surgery due to a tuberculum sellae meningioma that was wrapped around my pituitary gland and destroyed my optic nerve. I was diagnosed with hypothyroidism. My craniotomy surgery lasted twenty hours. I was in intensive care three days. I was weak and could not walk or even brush my teeth. I joined a support group eight months after surgery and began the protocol. I came into the Gary Null Running and Walking Club two months later and soon discontinued steroids, seizure pills, Synthroid, laxatives, and antacids. I no longer discuss my illness but speak of my health. I am naturally positive in thought, behavior, and speech. My physician does not understand my physical, emotional, and mental recovery in so short a time. I feel great and push forward without an attitude of handicap.

—Frank E.

Parkinson's Disease

My doctors had given up on me. They didn't tell me that, but I could see it in their eyes and hear it in their voices. They told me that I had Parkinson's and that there was no cure for it. They told me that Janet Reno and Muhammad Ali had forms of it and they were leading productive lives. This may sound strange, but the thing I feared the most about my condition was being unable to stop my shaking. This may sound selfish, but it is true. I visited Gary in his office on Seventy-second Street and Broadway, where he had me go to get my blood work done. Then he designed a program for me that changed my life. At first, I did not think I could go through with it. Now, I know I can. Although my shaking has not completely gone away, it has lessened a great deal. My wife is amazed at my progress, and I look forward to living the rest of my life knowing that one day, I will not be shaking at all.

—Joseph

Memory Loss

I was overjoyed to come into a Reversing the Aging support group. My memory was getting worse; I left my car keys in the trunk lock and my car was stolen. I was not organic but did juice and used supplements for a year before beginning the protocol.

Once I used organic produce and juice I began to feel stronger. I did not get sore throats since I began taking vitamin C at night. I decided to work less. A short time later I dated a man for the first time since my divorce eight years earlier. I felt happy and prayed for the return of my car. A short time later I spotted it while taking a long walk on an alternative trail. This increased my spiritual belief. I am building a cohesive relationship between my boyfriend, son, and myself. I sleep better, exercise, and work on an eating plan to prevent overeating.

—Virginia C.

Alzheimer's Disease

I am speaking for my wife, who gave me permission to do so. She is a little shy about these things, but she wants everyone to know her results. Two years ago she and I attended a lecture by Dr. Null. What he said gave us hope that my wife's Alzheimer's could be improved. We joined one of Gary's support groups and it has changed our lives. Alzheimer's runs in my wife's family. So, when she began forgetting things, we both suspected she had fallen victim to this dreaded disease. Her condition soon worsened, and her doctors could not give her anything to improve her condition. In Gary's support group, we completely changed our diets and began exercising. My wife said she could feel something like electricity in her brain that improved her memory and bettered her overall mood. People mistakenly believe that only one spouse gets a disease like Alzheimer's. This is not true. For when she got it, it affected me as well. Though she is not totally cured, she is a changed person. As a result, I am, too, a changed person.

—Egbert

Mental Fatigue

I had a "fuzzy" toxic head. I also had a lack of focus. The intensive focus on body-mind-spirit became clear in manifestation. I feel I have more focus and motivation and a new sense of who I am. My awareness is heightened. I believe I am moving toward divine health.

—Faye Marie L.

Headaches

I was diagnosed with a small melanoma in my right eye. I am legally blind in my left eye. The cancer options were horrendous: removing the eye, radiation, or leaving it with the chance it would metastasize to my liver. I often had migraine headaches, chronic lower back pain, prostate problems, a rotator cuff injury in my right shoulder, and arthritis in a toe. I was overweight. It was time to change strategies and rid myself of these conditions. Gary's words were powerful. I had to become my own authority. Since beginning the protocol the cancer has not grown for eight months. Migraine headaches virtually disappeared about two months after changing my diet, I lost thirty-five pounds, and my back has improved. Saw palmetto and other herbs did not relieve my prostate problem in the past, but they are quite effective now. My body is receptive to healing. The other minor conditions have improved. Although my energy level varies, I feel more energetic and younger in a body that knows how to heal itself.

—Eugene

Headaches

I suffered with bothersome tension-type headaches that sometimes became debilitating migraines. Since joining the group I am eating a primarily vegetarian diet including fish. I eliminated caffeine and sugar. I can state that I no longer have tension headaches. I feel very fortunate. I see changes in my physical health and awareness around me. Understanding my life energies further empowered me with insight and understanding.

—Natalie K.

Parkinson's Disease

I am a Parkinson's patient. I had hypertension, B-simplex outbreaks, and arthritis and skin problems. I became aware of the importance of nutrition and studied various theories, but my physical problems continued. Parkinson's symptoms caused me shame in public. I could not write and I typed with two fingers. My hands trembled when I put food in my mouth. I was prescribed medications, but past experiences were unpleasant so I refused them. I began Gary's detoxification protocol and learned the specifics of diet and organics, the biochemical necessity of green juices and grasses, the importance of attitude and beliefs. Things began to look up. I uncluttered my life of people and objects, and I now honor myself and share my knowledge with others. I am alert without past negative influences. These are my happiest and proudest times. I am seventy now and I intend to live another twenty years.

—Thomas

ENDNOTES

CHAPTER 1

1. E. Gould, A. J. Reeves, F. Mazyar, P. Tanapat, C. G. Gross, and E. Fuchs, "Hippocampal neurogenesis in adult Old World primates," *Neurobiology* 96, no. 9 (April 1999), pp. 5263–67.

2. Agency for Toxic Substances and Disease Registry 2003 CERCLA Priority List of Hazardous Substances; available online at www.atsdr.cdc.gov/clist.html.

3. John Carpi, "Stress: It's Worse than You Think," *Psychology Today*, January 1, 1996.

4. J. Douglas Bremner, *Does Stress Damage the Brain? Understanding Trauma-Related Disorders from a Neurological Perspective* (New York: W. W. Norton & Co., 2002).

5. *Stanford News* press release, "New studies of human brain show stress may shrink neurons," August 14, 1996; available online at www.Stanford.edu/dept/news/relaged/960814shrnkbrain.html.

6. Robert Sapolsky, *Why Zebras Don't Get Ulcers: An Updated Guide to Stress, Stress-Related Diseases, and Coping* (New York: W. H. Freeman, 1998).

7. *Diagnostic and Statistical Manual of Mental Disorders III, Revised (DSM-IV-R)*, code 219.00, Nicotine Withdrawal (Washington, D.C.: American Psychiatric Association, 1994).

8. Joel Fuhrman on *The Gary Null Show* on VoiceAmerica, November 11, 2004. Joel Fuhrman, M.D., is a board-certified family physician.

314//// APPENDICES

CHAPTER 2

1. J. Madeleine Nash, "Fertile Minds," *Time*, February 3, 1997.

2. Stephen Nohlgren, "Challenging, nurturing the brain keeps it healthy," *St. Petersburg Times*, March 13, 2005.

3. Lawrence C. Katz, Ph.D., *Keep Your Brain Alive* (New York: Workman Publishing, 1998).

4. J. Weuve, J. H. Kang, J. E. Manson, M. B. Breteler, J. Ware, and F. Grodstein, "Physical Activity, Including Walking, and Cognitive Function in Older Women," *JAMA* 292 (September 22–29, 2004), pp. 1454–61.

5. N. Scarmeas, G. Levy, M.-X. Tang, et al., "Influence of leisure activity on the incidence of Alzheimer's disease," *Neurology* 57 (2001), pp. 2236–42.

6. K. Yaffe, D. Barnes, M. Nevitt, L. Lui, and K. Covinsky, "A Prospective Study of Physical Activity and Cognitive Decline in Elderly Women: Women Who Walk," *Archives of Internal Medicine* 161 (July 23, 2001), pp. 1703–08.

7. American Association of Retired Persons (AARP), "Let's Dance to Health"; available online at www.aarp.org/health/fitness/get_motivated/lets_dance_to_health.html.

8. Yaffe et al., "A Prospective Study of Physical Activity."

9. "Longevity—A Challenge for the Individual and the Society." Speech by Ursula Lehr, Ph.D., May 18, 2000, Colegio de Medicos de Madrid; available online at http://www.segg.es/segg/html/socios/formacion_continuada/casos_clinicas/lehr.htm.

10. Marc Kaufman, "Meditation Gives Brain a Charge, Study Finds," *Washington Post*, January 3, 2005, p. A05; available online at www.washingtonpost.com/wp-dyn/articles/243006-2005Jan2.html.

11. Ibid.

12. P. C. Bickford et al., "Diets high in antioxidants can reverse age-related declines in cerebellar beta-adrenergic receptor functions and motor learning." Paper presented at the 1999 AGE Annual Meeting, Seattle; and L. Buee, "Cerebrovascular aging," *Therapie* 54 (1999), pp. 155–65.

13. News Release from *Journal of Experimental Medicine*, March 14, 2005, "Eating Oily Fish May Reduce Inflammation"; available online at www.sciencedaily.com.

14. A. M. al-Awadhi, C. D. Dunn, "Effects of fish-oil constituents and plasma lipids on fibrinolysis in vitro," *British Journal of Biomedical Science* 57, no. 4 (2000), pp. 273–80.

15. "Fish Oil Holds Promise in Alzheimer's Fight," May 29, 2005. Press release from U.S. Department of Veterans Affairs, Washington, D.C.; available online at www.sciencedaily.com.

16. S. M. Loriaux, J. B. Deijen, J. F. Oriebeke, and J. H. De Swart, "The effects of nicotinic acid and xanthinol nicotinate on human memory in different categories of age. A double blind study," *Psychopharmacology* (Berl) 87, no. 4 (1985), pp. 390–95.

17. J. E. Alpert, M. Fava, "Nutrition and depression: the role of folate," *Nutrition Review* 55, no. 5 (May 1997), pp. 145–49.

18. Marc Kaufman, "Meditation Gives Brain a Charge, Study Finds," *The Washington Post,* January 3, 2005.

19. J. Areart-Treichel, "Nutrient Combo Boosts Memory—At Least in Rats," *Psychiatric News* 37, no. 8 (April 2002), p. 58.

20. Ibid.

21. R. P. Ostrowski, "Effect of coenzyme Q10 (coQ10) on superoxide dismutase activity in ET-1 and ET-3 experimental models of cerebral ischemia in the rat," *Folia Neuropathology* 37, no. 4 (1999), pp. 247–51.

22. M. E. Rhodes, P.-K. Li, J. F. Flood, and D. A. Johnson, "Enhancement of hippocampal acetylcholine release by the neurosteroid dehydroepiandrosterone sulfate: An in vivo microdialysis study," *Brain Research* 733 (1996), pp. 284–86.

23. T. Maurice et al., "Dehydroepiandrosterone sulfate attenuates dizocilpine-induced learning impairment in mice via sigma 1- receptors," *Behavioral Brain Research* 83, no. 1–2 (February 1997), pp. 159–64.

24. H. D. Danenboerg et al., "Dehydroepiandrosterone (DHEA) increases production and release of Alzheimer's amyloid precursor protein," *Life Science* 59, no. 19 (1996), pp. 1651–57.

25. H. Nagasawa, K. Kogure, K. Kawashima, et al., "Effects of co-dergocrine mesylate (hydergine) in multi-infarct dementia as evaluated by positron emission tomography," *Tohoku Journal of Experimental Medicine* 162, no. 3 (November 1990), pp. 225–33.

26. M. Ditch, F. J. Kelly, and O. Resnick, "An ergot preparation (hydergine) in the treatment of cerebrovascular disorders in the geriatric patient: double blind study," *Journal of the American Geriatric Society* 19, no. 3 (March 1971), pp. 208–17.

27. H. Emmenegger, W. Meier-Ruge, "The actions of hydergine on the brain. A histochemical, circulatory and neurophysical study," *Pharmacology* 1, no. 1 (1968), pp. 65–78.

28. P. M. Kidd, "A review of nutrients and botanicals in the integrative management of cognitive dysfunction," *Alternative Medicine Review* 4, no. 3 (June 1999), pp. 144–61.

29. P. J. Delwaide et al., "Double-blind randomized controlled study of phosphatidylserine in senile demented patients," *Acta Neurological Scandinavica* 73, no. 2 (February 1986), pp. 136–40.

30. D. Bagchi, R. L. Krohn, M. Bagchi, et al., "Oxygen free radical scavenging abilities of vitamins C and E, and a grape seed proanthocyanidin extract in vitro," *Research Communications in Molecular Pathology and Pharmacology* 95 (1997), pp. 179–89.

31. P. Jones, D. Takai, "The Role of DNA Methylation in Mammalian Epigenesis," *Science* (August 10, 2001), pp. 1068–70.

CHAPTER 3

1. From HealthyPlace.com, "Depression in Elderly"; available online at www.healthyplace.com/communities/depression/elderly.asp.

2. Ricki Lewis, Ph.D., "Evening out the Ups and Downs of Manic-Depressive Illness," *FDA Consumer Magazine*, June 1996.

3. Dr. Ronald M. Podell, *Contagious Emotions: Staying Well When Your Loved One Is Depressed* (New York: Pocket Books, 1993).

4. Dr. Lewis Harrison on *The Gary Null Show* on VoiceAmerica, November 30, 2004.

5. Ibid.

6. T. L. Brink, J. A. Yesavage, O. Lum, P. Heersema, M. B. Adey, and T. L. Rose, "Screening tests for geriatric depression," *Clinical Gerontologist* 1 (1982), pp. 37–44; see also J. A. Yesavage, T. L. Brink, T. L. Rose, O. Lum, V. Huang, M. B. Adey, and V. O. Leirer, "Development and validation of a geriatric depression scale: A preliminary report," *Journal of Psychiatric Research* 17 (1983), pp. 37–49; and J. I. Sheikh, J. A. Yesavage, J. O. Brooks III, L. F. Friedman, P. Gratzinger, R. D. Hill, A. Zadeik, and T. Crook, "Proposed factor structure of the Geriatric Depression Scale," *International Psychogeriatrics* 3 (1991), pp. 23–28.

7. R. C. Casper, "Nutrients, neurodevelopment, and mood," *Current Psychiatry Report* 6, no. 6 (December 2004), pp. 425–29.

8. J. E. Alpert, M. Fava, "Nutrition and Depression: the role of folate," *Nutrition Review* 55, no. 5 (May 1977), pp. 145–49.

9. D. Frizel et al., "Plasma magnesium and calcium in depression," *British Journal of Psychiatry* 115 (1969), pp. 1275–77.

10. H. Beckman, M. A. Strauss, and E. Ludolph, "DL-Phenylalanine in depressed patients: an open study," *Journal of Neural Transmission* 41 (1977), pp. 123–34.

11. K. D. Hansgen, J. Vesper, and M. Ploch, "Multi-center double-blind study examining the antidepressant effectiveness of the Hypericum extract LI 160," *Journal of Geriatric Psychiatry and Neurology* 7, supp. 1 (1994), pp. 15–18.

12. H. Schubet, P. Halam, "Depressive episode primarily unresponsive to therapy in elderly patients. Efficacy of ginkgo biloba extract (EGb 761) in combination with antidepressants," *Geriatric Forschung* 3 (1993), pp. 45–53.

13. Michael J. Norden, M.D., *Beyond Prozac: Brain-Toxic Lifestyles, Natural Antidotes & New Generation Antidepressants* (New York: Regan Books, 1995).

CHAPTER 4

1. Richard Restak, M.D., on *The Gary Null Show* on VoiceAmerica, November 24, 2004. Restak is a preeminent neuropsychiatrist and author of several books, including *The New Brain: How the Modern Age Is Rewiring Your Mind* (New York: Rodale, 2003).

2. *The Gary Null Show* on VoiceAmerica, November 24, 2004. Data taken from W. E. Narrow, D. S. Rae, D. A. Regier, "NIMH epidemiology note: prevalence of anxiety disorders. Population estimates based on U.S. Census estimated residential population age 18 to 54 on July 1, 1998." Unpublished.

3. "Anxiety: Should You Let It Worry You?"; available online at www.pdrhealth.com.

4. *Merck Manual of Geriatrics*, 3rd ed., chap. 34, "Anxiety Disorders" (Whitehouse Station, N.J.: Merck Research Laboratories, Division of Merck & Co., Inc., 2000).

5. From Epidemiologic Cachement Area Study conducted by NIH in 1996.

6. L. N. Robins, D. A. Regier, eds., *Psychiatric Disorders in America: the Epidemiologic Cachement Area Study* (New York: The Free Press, 1991).

7. Anxiety Disorders Association of America Web site, www.adaa.org, adapted from A. J. Land, Ph.D., and M. B. Stein, M.D., "Anxiety Disorders: How to Recognize and Treat the Medical Symptoms of Emotional Illness," *Geriatrics* 56, no. 5 (May 2001), pp. 24–27, 31–34.

8. Norman Brown, "Do you suffer high anxiety? Research reveals more about how stress affects body and mind. Here is the rundown on causes and therapies," *VFW Magazine*, January 2003.

9. Ibid.

10. D. S. Charney, G. R. Heninger, and P. I. Jatlow, "Increased axiogenic effects of caffeine in panic disorders," *Archives of General Psychiatry* 42, no. 3 (March 1985), pp. 233–43.

11. J. P. Boulenger, T. W. Uhde, E. A. Wolff III, and R. M. Post, "Increased sensitivity to caffeine in patients with panic disorders. Preliminary evidence," *Archives of General Psychiatry* 41, no. 11 (November 1984), pp. 1067–71.

12. M. Y. Geng, H. Saito, and N. Nishiyama, "Protective effects of pyridoxal phosphate against glucose deprivation-induced damage in cultured hippocampal neurons," *Journal of Neurochemistry* 68, no. 6 (June 1997), pp. 2500–06.

13. R. A. Akhundov, V. V. Rozhanets, T. A. Voronina, and A. V. Valdman, "Mechanism of the tranquilizing action of electron structural analogs of nicotinamide," Biull Eksp Biol Med. 101, no. 3 (March 1986), pp. 329–31.

14. A. Palatnik, K. Frolov, M. Fux, and J. Benjamin, "Double-blind, controlled, crossover trial of inositol versus fluvoxamine for the treatment of panic disorder," *Journal of Clinical Psychopharmacology* 21, no. 3 (June 2001), pp. 335–39.

15. K. D. Hansgen, J. Vesper, and M. Ploch, "Multi-center double-blind study examining the antidepressant effectiveness of the Hypericum extract LI 160."

16. T. Field, "Massage therapy effects," *American Psychologist* 53, no. 12 (1998), pp. 1270–81.

17. Stephanie Marohn on *The Gary Null Show* on VoiceAmerica, November 22, 2004. Marohn is a writer and editor of books on psychospirituality and alternative thought.

CHAPTER 5

1. Paul Scheele on *The Gary Null Show* on VoiceAmerica, November 29, 2004. Scheele is the founder of Learning Strategies Corporation.

2. Ibid.

3. Dr. Dharma Singh Khalsa on *The Gary Null Show* on VoiceAmerica, November 26, 2004. Dr. Singh Khalsa is President and Medical Director of the Alzheimer's Prevention Foundation International in Tucson, Arizona.

4. "Staying Sharp, Memory Loss and Aging," 2004 AARP Foundation and the Dana Alliance for Brain Initiatives.

5. T. D. Smith, M. M. Adams, M. Gallagher, J. H. Morrison, and P. R. Rapp, "Circuit-specific alterations in hippocampal synaptophysin immunoreactivity predict spatial learning impairment in aged rats," *Journal of Neuroscience* 20, no. 17 (September 2000), pp. 6578–93.

6. A. D. Mooradian, "Effect of aging on the blood-brain barrier," *Neurobiology of Aging* 9, no. 1 (January–February 1988), pp. 31–39.

7. Elisa Lottor, Ph.D., ND, and Nancy Bruning, *Female and Forgetful: A Six-Step Program to Help Restore Your Memory and Sharpen Your Mind* (New York: Warner Books, 2002).

8. C. Decarle, B. L. Miller, G. E. Swan, et al., "Predictors of brain morphology for the men of the NHLBI twin study," *Stroke* 30, no. 3 (March 1999), pp. 529–36.

9. J. S. Rhodes, H. van Praag, S. Jeffrey, I. Girard, G. S. Mitchell, T. Garland Jr., and F. H. Gage, "Exercise increases hippocampal neurogenesis to high levels but does not improve spatial learning in mice bred for increased voluntary wheel running," *Behavioral Neuroscience* 117, no. 5 (October 2003), pp. 1006–16.

10. Gary Null with Dr. Dharma Singh Khalsa, "Improving Memory Function," November 26, 2004.

11. R. G. Thompson, C. J. Moulin, S. Hayre, and R. W. Jones, "Music enhances category fluency in healthy older adults and Alzheimer's disease patients," *Experimental Aging Research* 31, no. 1 (January–March 2005), pp. 91–99.

12. B. Draganski, C. Gaser, V. Busch, G. Schuierer, U. Bogdahn, and A. May, "Neuroplasticity: Changes in grey matter induced by training," *Nature* 427 (January 22, 2005), pp. 311–12.

13. M. C. Morris, D. A. Evans, J. L. Bienias, C. C. Tangney, and R. S. Wilson, "Vitamin E and cognitive decline in older persons," *Archives of Neurology* 59, no. 7 (July 2002), pp. 1125–32.

14. Ibid.

15. M. S. Morris, P. F. Jacques, I. H. Rosenberg, and J. Selhub, "National Health and Nutrition Examination Survey: Hyperhomocysteinemia associated with poor recall in the third National Health and Nutrition Examination Survey," *American Journal of Clinical Nutrition* 73, no. 5 (May 2001), pp. 927–33.

16. H. P. Volz, U. Hehnke, and W. Hauke, "Improvement in quality of life in the elderly. Results of a placebo-controlled study on the efficacy and tolerability of lecithin fluid in patients with impaired cognitive functions," *MMW Fortschr Medicine* 146 (December 9, 2004), pp. 99–106.

17. P. M. Kidd, "A review of nutrients and botanicals in the integrative management of cognitive dysfunction," *Alternative Medicine Review* 4, no. 3 (June 1999), pp. 144–61.

CHAPTER 6

1. S. Kaplan, "The restorative benefits of nature: Toward an integrative framework," Special Issue: Green Psychology, *Journal of Environmental Psychology* 15, no. 3 (1995), pp. 169–82.

2. Edward O. Wilson, *Biophilia: The Human Bond with Other Species* (Cambridge: Harvard University Press, (reprint) 1986).

3. Annual Meeting of the Society of Psychophysiological Research in Montreal, Canada, October 1981.

4. A. Watanabe et al., "Effects of creatine on mental fatigue and cerebral hemoglobin oxygenation," *Euroscience Research* 42, no. 4 (April 2002), pp. 279–85.

5. V. Darbinyan, A. Kteyan, A. Panossian, E. Gabrielian, G. Wikman, and H. Wagner, "Rhodiola rosea in stress-induced fatigue—a double-blind crossover study of a standardized extract SHR-5 with a repeated low-dose regimen on the mental performance of healthy physicians during night duty," *Phytomedicine* 7 (2000), pp. 365–71.

6. A. A. Spasov, G. K. Wikman, V. B. Mandrikov, I. A. Mironova, and V. V. Neumoin, "A double-blind, placebo-controlled pilot study of the stimulating and adaptogenic effect of Rhodiola rosea SHR-5 extract on the fatigue of students caused by stress during an examination period with a repeated low-dose regimen," *Phytomedicine* 7 (2000), pp. 85–89.

CHAPTER 7

1. E. Mohr, T. Mendis, and J. D. Grimes, "Late cognitive changes in Parkinson's disease with an emphasis on dementia," *Advances in Neurology* 65 (1995), pp. 97–113.

2. In their search for an electron to pair with a free radical, atoms inflict damage on their donor atoms. The result ultimately damages the cells throughout the body, including those of the brain. Metals like iron, copper, and

aluminum accelerate the free radical chain of reaction, producing excessive amounts of these metals in the brains of Parkinson's sufferers.

3. Joan Stephenson, Ph.D., "Exposure to Home Pesticides Linked to Parkinson's Disease," *JAMA* 283 (2000), pp. 3055–56.

4. P. C. Holland, J. S. Han, and M. Gallagher, "Lesions of the amygdala central nucleus alter performance on a selective attention task," *Journal of Neuroscience* 20, no. 17 (September 1, 2000), pp. 6701–06.

5. From the Web site of The National Parkinson's Foundation.

6. D. E. Riley, "Secondary Parkinsonism," in *Parkinson's Disease and Movement Disorders*, 3rd ed., edited by J. Jankovic and E. Tolosa (New York: LW&W, 1998), pp. 317–28.

7. A. J. Hughes, S. E. Daniel, L. Kilford, and A. J. Lees, "Accuracy of clinical diagnosis of idiopathic Parkinson's disease: a clinico-pathological study of 100 cases," *Journal of Neurology, Neurosurgery, and Psychiatry* 55, no. 3 (March 1992), pp. 181–84.

8. A. I. Tröster, J. A. Fields, and W. C. Koller, "Parkinson's disease and Parkinsonism," in *Textbook of Geriatric Neuropsychiatry*, 2nd ed., edited by C. E. Coffey and J. L. Cummings (Washington, D.C.: American Psychiatric Press, 2000), p. 562.

9. J. R. Chacon, E. Duran, J. A. Duran, et al., "Usefulness of olanzopine in the levodopa-induced psychosis in patients with Parkinson's disease," *Neurologia* 17, no. 1 (January 2002), pp. 7–11.

10. C. W. Olanow, P. Jenner, N. Tatton, and W. Tatton, "Neurodegeneration and Parkinson's disease," in *Parkinson's Disease and Movement Disorders*, 3rd ed., edited by J. Jankovic and E. Tolosa (New York: LW&W, 1998), pp. 67–103.

11. S. Fahn, "An open trial of high-dosage antioxidants in early Parkinson's disease," *American Journal of Clinical Nutrition* 53, supp. 1 (January 1991), pp. S380–82.

12. W. Hellenbrand, H. Boeing, B. P. Robra, et al., "Diet and Parkinson's disease. II: A possible role for the past intake of specific nutrients. Results from a self-administered food-frequency questionnaire in a case-control study," *Neurology* 47, no. 3 (September 1996), pp. 644–50.

13. M. Ebadi, J. F. Rodriguez-Sierra, and N. S. Norton, "Glutathione and Metallothionein in Neurodegeneration—Neuroprotection of Parkinson's Disease," *NEL* 18, no. 2–3 (1998), pp. 111–22.

14. "Jefferson researchers show melatonin's potential benefits in preventing Parkinson's damage." Press release from Thomas Jefferson Medical College

at Thomas Jefferson University, Philadelphia, PA, October 24, 1999; available online at www.mult-sclerosis.org/news/Oct1999/MelatoninParkinsons .html.

15. D. Bagchi, R. L. Krohn, M. Bagchi, et al., "Oxygen free radical scavenging abilities of vitamins C and E."

CHAPTER 8

1. Statistics taken from Alzheimer's Association; available online at www.alz .org/AboutAD/Statistics.asp.

2. Adapted from The Alzheimer's Information Site; available online at www.alzinfo.org.

3. Ibid.

4. Adapted from Administration on Aging Alzheimer's Disease Info; available online at www.aoa.gov/ALZ/Public/alzcarefam/disease_info/questions_ to_ask_pf.asp.

5. Alzheimer's Association International Conference on Prevention of Dementia, June 18–21, 2005, Washington, D.C.; available online at www.alz.org/ preventionconference/pc2005/.

6. "Exercise Slows Development of Alzheimer's-Like Brain Changes in Mice, New Study Finds," *NIH News*, April 25, 2005.

7. J. Verghese, R. B. Lipton, M. J. Katz, C. B. Hall, C. A. Derby, G. Kuslansky, A. F. Ambrose, M. Sliwinski, and H. Buschke, "Leisure Activities and the Risk of Dementia in the Elderly," *New England Journal of Medicine* 348, no. 25 (2003), pp. 2508–16.

8. P. E. Newman, "Could diet be one of the causal factors of Alzheimer's disease?" *Medical Hypotheses* 39, no. 2 (1992), pp. 123–26.

9. S. Yehuda, S. Rabinovitz, et al., "Essential fatty acids preparation (SR-3) improves Alzheimer's patients' quality of life," *International Journal of Neuroscience* 87, no. 3–4 (1996), pp.141–49.

10. M. Sano, C. Ernesto, et al., "A controlled trial of selegiline, alpha-tocopherol, or both as treatment for Alzheimer's disease: The Alzheimer's Disease Cooperative Study," *New England Journal of Medicine* 336, no. 17 (1997), pp. 1216–22.

11. P. M. Kidd, "A review of nutrients and botanicals in the integrative management of cognitive dysfunction," *Alternative Medicine Review* 4, no. 3 (June 1999), pp. 144–61.

12. P. L. Le Bars, M. M. Katz, N. Berman, et al., "A placebo-controlled, double-blind, randomized trial of an extract of ginkgo biloba for dementia," *JAMA* 278, no. 16 (1997), pp. 1327–32.

13. Q. Wang, K. Iwasaki, T. Suzuki, H. Arai, Y. Ikarashi, T. Yabe, K. Toriizuka, T. Hanawa, H. Yamada, and H. Sasaki, "Potentiation of brain acetylcholine neurons by Kami-Untan-To (KUT) in aged mice: implications for a possible antidementia drug," *Phytomedicine* 7, no. 4 (July 2000), pp. 253–58.

14. H. Arai, T. Suzuki, H. Sasaki, T. Hanawa, K. Toriizuka, and H. Yamada, "A new interventional strategy for Alzheimer's disease by Japanese herbal medicine," *Nippon Ronen Igakkai Zasshi* 37, no. 3 (March 2000), pp. 212–15.

15. S. S. Xu, Z. X. Goa, Z. Weng, et al., "Efficacy of tablet huperzine-A on memory, cognition and behavior in Alzheimer's disease," *Chung kUo Yao Li Hsueh Pao* 16 (1995), pp. 391–95.

CHAPTER 9

1. J. P. Boulenger, T. W. Uhde, E. A. Wolff III, and R. M. Post, "Increased sensitivity to caffeine."

2. A. Mauskop, B. M. Altura, "Role of magnesium in the pathogenesis and treatment of migraines," *Clinical Neuroscience* 5, no. 1 (1998), pp. 24–27.

3. A. Peikert et al., "Prophylaxis of Migraine with Oral Magnesium: Results from a prospective multi-center, placebo-controlled and double-blind randomized study," *Cephalagia* 16 (1996), pp. 257–63.

4. B. Claustrat, J. Brun, M. Geoffriau, R. Zaidan, C. Mallo, and G. Chazot, "Nocturnal plasma melatonin profile and melatonin kinetics during infusion in status migrainosus," *Cephalagia* 17, no. 4 (June 1997), pp. 511–17.

5. T. Field, "Massage therapy effects," *American Psychologist* 53, no. 12 (1998), pp. 1270–81.

CHAPTER 10

1. Scott Shepherd, M. D., "Head Trauma," August 20, 2004; available online at www.emedicine.com.

2. S. Moochhala, J. Lu, "Potential use of stem cell therapy for traumatic brain injury," Defence Medical & Environmental Research Institute, 117510. DSO National Laboratories, Singapore.

3. J. H. Bower, D. M. Maraganore, B. J. Peterson, "Head trauma preceding PD," *Neurology* 60 (2003), pp. 1610–15.

4. D. Shoumitro, I. Lyons, M. Koutzoukis, I. Ali, and G. McCarthy, "Rate of psychiatric illness 1 year after traumatic brain injury," *American Journal of Psychiatry* 156 (March 1999), pp. 374–78.

5. James M. Connor, Andrea A. Chiba, and Mark H. Tuszynski, "The Basal Forebrain Cholinergic System Is Essential for Cortical Plasticity and Functional Recovery Following Brain Injury," *Neuron* 46, no. 2 (April 21, 2005), pp. 173–79.

6. F. Yang, G. P. Lim, A. N. Begum, O. J. Ubeda, M. R. Simmons, S. S. Ambegaokar, P. P. Chen, R. Kayed, C. G. Glabe, S. A. Frautschy, and G. M. Cole, "Curcumin inhibits formation of A oligomers and fibrils and binds plaques and reduces amyloid in vivo," *Journal of Biological Chemistry* 280, no. 7 (February 18, 2005), pp. 5892–5901.

7. Joie Guner, "The Curry Cure," *UCLA Daily Bruin Online,* January 14, 2005.

8. P. J. O'Connor, N. P. Pronk, A. Tan, and R. R. Whitebird, "Characteristics of adults who use prayer as an alternative therapy," *American Journal of Health Promotion* 19, no. 5 (May–June 2005), pp. 369–75.

9. R. F. Palmer, D. Katerndahl, J. Morgan-Kidd, "A randomized trial of the effects of remote intercessory prayer: interactions with personal beliefs on problem-specific outcomes and functional status," *Journal of Alternative and Complementary Medicine* 10, no. 3 (June 2004), pp. 438–48.

CHAPTER 12

1. K. D. Hansgen, J. Vesper, and M. Ploch, "Multi-center double-blind study examining the antidepressant effectiveness of the Hypericum extract LI 160."

2. T. Field, "Massage therapy effects."

CHAPTER 13

1. D. S. Knopman, S. T. DeKosky, J. L. Cummings, et al., "Practice parameter: Diagnosis of dementia (an evidence-based review)." Report of the Quality Standards Subcommittee of the American Academy of Neurology. *Neurology* 56 (2001), pp. 1143–53.

2. Adapted from Administration on Aging Alzheimer's Disease Info; available online at www.aoa.gov/ALZ/Public/alzcarefam/disease_info/questions_to_ask_pf.asp.

3. Alzheimer's Association International Conference on Prevention of Dementia, June 18–21, 2005, Washington, D.C.; available online at www.alz.org/preventionconference/pc2005/.

4. "Exercise Slows Development of Alzheimer's-Like Brain Changes in Mice, New Study Finds," *NIH News*, April 25, 2005.

5. J. Verghese et al., "Leisure Activities and the Risk of Dementia in the Elderly."

6. R. A. Whitmer, E. P. Gunderson, E. Barrett-Connor, C. P. Quesenberry, and K. Yaffe, "Obesity in middle age and future risk of dementia: a 27-year longitudinal population-based study," *BJM*, doi:10.1136/bmj.384446.466238.EO (published April 29, 2005).

7. M. Sano, C. Ernesto, et al., "A controlled trial of selegiline, alpha-tocopherol, or both as treatment for Alzheimer's disease."

8. P. M. Kidd, "A review of nutrients and botanicals in the integrative management of cognitive dysfunction."

9. P. L. Le Bars et al., "A placebo-controlled, double-blind, randomized trial of an extract of ginkgo biloba for dementia."

10. Q. Wang et al., "Potentiation of brain acetylcholine neurons by Kami-Untan-To (KUT) in aged mice: implications for a possible antidementia drug."

11. H. Arai et al., "A new interventional strategy for Alzheimer's disease by Japanese herbal medicine."

12. S. S. Xu et al., "Efficacy of tablet huperzine-A on memory, cognition and behavior in Alzheimer's disease."

CHAPTER 14

1. C. B. Pert, S. H. Snyder, "Opiate receptor: demonstration in nervous tissue," *Science* 179, no. 77 (March 1973), pp. 1011–14.

2. Irving Kirsch and Guy Sapirstein, "Listening to Prozac but Hearing Placebo: A Meta-Analysis of Antidepressant Medication," *Prevention & Treatment* 1 (June 1998), article 0002a.

3. S. F. Maier and L. R. Watkins, "Cytokines for psychologists: implications of bidirectional immune-to-brain communication for understanding behavior, mood, and cognition," *Psychological Review* 105 (1998), pp. 83–107.

4. S. E. Hammack, K. J. Richey, L. R. Watkins, and S. F. Maier, "The role of corticotropin releasing hormone in the dorsal raphe nucleus in mediating the behavioral consequences of uncontrollable stress," *Journal of Neuroscience* 22 (2002), pp. 1020–26.

5. Marc Barasch, "Welcome to the Mind-Body Revolution," *Psychology Today*, July/August 1996.

6. G. F. Soloman, "The emerging field of psychoneuroimmunology," *Advances* 2, no. 1 (1985), pp. 6–19.

7. S. F. Maier and L. R. Watkins, "Cytokines for psychologists."

8. K. A. O'Connor, J. D. Johnson, M. K. Hansen, Frank J. L. Wieseler, E. Maksimova, L. R. Watkins, and S. F. Maier, "Peripheral and central proinflammatory cytokine response to a severe acute stressor," *Brain Research* 991, no. 1–2 (November 21, 2003), pp. 123–32.

9. Ibid.

10. Beth Azar, "A new take on psychoneuroimmunology," *Monitor on Psychology* 32, no. 11 (December 2001).

11. See Herbert Benson's *The Relaxation Response* (New York: Avon Books, 1975), and *Beyond the Relaxation Response* (New York: Berkley Books, 1985).

12. Andrew Weil, M.D., *Spontaneous Healing* (New York: Ballantine Books, 1996).

13. Lauran Neergaard, "Brain Exercise Is Key to Healthy Mind," Associated Press, June 20, 2005.

14. Kathy Facklemann, "Lifestyle link to Alzheimer's strengthens," *USA Today*, June 19, 2005.

15. David M. Nathan, M.D., and Linda Delahanty, M.S., R.D., "Better Ways to Beat Diabetes," *Newsweek*, Summer 2005.